In the Trenches: A Young

Physician's Odyssey

By

Queeneth Adams

© Copyright 2024 by Queeneth Adams

All rights reserved.

No part of this book may be reproduced, stored in a retrieval system, or transmitted, in any form or by any means, electronic, mechanical, photocopying, recording, or otherwise, without prior written permission from the publisher, except for brief quotations embodied in critical reviews and certain other noncommercial uses permitted by copyright law.

ISBN:

[9798340868473]

With love and gratitude, I dedicate this book to God, my heavenly father, who has guided my path and inspired my heart.

And to my parents, Prince Ekpo Effiwatt and Princess Winifred Effiwatt, who nurtured my dreams and encouraged me to pursue them.

Acknowledgment

I would like to extend my heartfelt gratitude to my loving family, without whom this book would not have been possible.

To my husband, Hon. Richard Adams, thank you for believing in me and for being my partner in every sense of the word.

To my beautiful children, Eden, Elyon, and Richard Jr., you are my inspiration and my joy. Your love and enthusiasm have kept me going even on the toughest of days. I am so proud to be your parent and to have had the opportunity to share this experience with you. Thank you all for your patience, understanding, and love. This book is as much yours as it is mine.

My sincere gratitude to my senior colleagues/instructors, Dr Elvis Bisong and Dr Abraham Gyuse for their invaluable contributions in this book.

Preface

Starting my medical career in Nigeria was a mixed bag of emotions – exhilarating and daunting. The satisfaction of graduating from medical school after years of hard work was tempered by the sobering realization that I was now responsible for real human lives, not just textbooks, lab samples, or cadavers.

However, nothing could have prepared me for the unspoken challenges of practicing medicine in an under-resourced setting. I faced numerous obstacles, including:

- Unavailable or faulty medical equipment
- Scarce public amenities
- Financial hardship among patients, exacerbated by the lack of healthcare insurance
- Unfavorable local culture and traditions that clashed with orthodox medical practice
- Superstitious beliefs

During my Family Medicine residency, I encountered many patients who left an indelible mark on me. This book is a collection of remarkable cases that had a profound impact on my growth as a physician. Through these stories, I share the lessons I learned and highlight the struggles faced by physicians in underdeveloped settings.

Despite the limitations, these healthcare providers are just as vital to their communities as their peers in better-resourced settings.

Contents

Chapter One 1
Allergic Conjunctivitis In A Primary School Child 1

Chapter Two 17
External Hordeolum In A Make-Up Artist 17

Chapter Three... 33
Recurrent Pelvic Inflammatory Disease In A 28-Year-Old Woman With Multiple Sexual Partners 33

Chapter Four... 52
Septic Abortion In A High School Student 52

Chapter Five 71
Malaria In Pregnancy 71

Chapter Six 87
Retained Placenta In A 31-Year-Old Woman 87

Chapter Seven... 104
Foreign Body In The Ear 104

Chapter Eight.. 120
Chronic Leg Ulcer Due To Varicose Veins 120

Chapter Nine... 140
Left Dorsal Wrist Ganglion In A 28-Year-Old Woman ... 140

Chapter Ten... 156
Severe Hypertension Due To Poor Adherence 156

Chapter Eleven 175
Urinary Tract Infection In A 33-Year-Old Woman With An Ectopic Kidney 175

Chapter Twelve 193
Food Poisoning In A Nurse 193

Chapter Thirteen 207
Vaso-Occlusive Crisis In A 7-Year-Old Sickler 207

Chapter Fourteen 225
Scabies In A 13-Year-Old Student 225

Chapter Fifteen 241
Acute Tonsillopharyngitis In A 10-Year-Old Boy 241

Chapter Sixteen 257
Cervical Spondylosis In A 70-Year-Old Woman 257

Chapter Seventeen 273
Depression Following Burns Injury In A Welder 273

Chapter Eighteen 289
Post-Traumatic Stress Disorder Following Intimate Partner Violence In A Female Civil Servant 289

Chapter Nineteen 306
The Importance Of Adequate Counselling In The Family Planning Clinic 306

Chapter Twenty 319
The Effect Of Sexual Assault On The Family 319

Page Left Blank Intentionally

Chapter One

Allergic Conjunctivitis In A Primary School Child

A nine-year-old boy presented to the clinic with itching, redness, and swelling of the eyes for 2 days' duration. He was apparently well until two days prior to the presentation, when he developed intense itching in both eyes. The itching was continuous and associated with a watery discharge. There was redness and slight swelling of both eyes, which had developed as the patient vigorously rubbed his eyes. He also complained of a sandy sensation in his eyes.

There was no eye pain, no blurring of vision, or inability to see; however, the symptoms were so distressing that they prevented him from sleeping properly at night, reading, and doing his homework. There was no history of trauma or contact with any person who had an eye discharge and no history of a urethral discharge. There was a history of catarrh and cough, which had occurred a week earlier. There was a history of similar eye symptoms which had occurred twice within the previous year. He developed pruritic rashes anytime he consumed milk and groundnuts. This is usually resolved by the consumption of Phenergan syrup. He was allergic to dust and woolen materials. On waking up most mornings, he sneezed continuously and had a runny nose, which usually cleared as the day progressed. There was a positive family history of asthma as his deceased paternal grandfather, two paternal aunts, one paternal uncle, and three paternal cousins all had asthma.

His mother felt that his current symptoms were due to an infection from school and feared that since the eye symptoms were recurrent, they would gravely impact his performance in the upcoming State Common Entrance exams as he was unable to concentrate on his studies. As such, he needed urgent medical intervention to bring a lasting solution.

His pregnancy was planned and uneventful. He was delivered to term; his birth weight was 3.7kg, and he cried at birth. His developmental milestones were normal for his age. He received all immunizations required by the National Program on Immunization, and this was evident on his immunization card. He had been admitted for pneumonia and generalized itchy skin rash in the past year. He had no history of surgical operations or transfusions.

He had been receiving Phenergan syrup intermittently for durations of 1 or more weeks to prevent body itching. This was self-medicated and not prescribed by a physician. His allergy history was outlined in the body of history. He was the 2nd child in a family of 3 children and was a Primary 5 pupil in a private school. His parents were both civil servants, and they lived in a 3-bedroom apartment. Both parents were non-smokers and did not drink alcohol. The family was at Stage 4 (family with school-age children) of Evelyn Duvall's family staging. Their family APGAR was scored as 8/10, showing a highly functional family, and the source of healthcare financing was out-of-pocket.

There was no history of throat pain, difficulty in swallowing, ear pain or discharge, chest pain, abdominal pain, or pain while urinating.

A physical examination showed an apparently healthy-looking male child. He had peri-orbital oedema in both eyes. The patient was afebrile, anicteric, and not cyanotic. He was neither pale nor dehydrated.

There was no lymph node enlargement or pedal oedema. His anthropometric parameters were normal for his age, with a weight being 34 kg and a height of 1.35cm. His visual acuity was 6/6 in both eyes, showing normal vision, and vision was preserved in all eye fields. The eyelids were swollen, and the conjunctivae were hyperemic. A strand of eyelash was present in the right conjunctiva. No discharge was seen on the eyelids. The right and left corneas were transparent, the anterior chambers had normal depth, and both pupils were symmetrical and reactive to light. Normal red reflexes were elicited in both eyes, and the retina was normal.

He was conscious and well-oriented. There was no evidence of meningeal irritation or cranial nerve deficit. Muscle tone, power, and reflexes were normal. His pulse rate was 94 beats per minute, regular and full volume. There was synchrony of the peripheral pulses. The blood pressure was 110/80mmHg. The first and second heart sounds were only heard. His respiratory rate was 14 cycles per minute. There was equal chest expansion, and breath sounds were vesicular. His abdomen was flat, soft, and moved with respiration. There was no tender area and no organomegaly. His bowel sounds were normoactive.

A provisional diagnosis of allergic conjunctivitis was made with a differential diagnosis of acute viral conjunctivitis.

Management:

The diagnosis and management plan were fully explained to the patient and his mother. They were told that the condition was most likely due to an allergic state, and not passed on to the patient by contact, as was believed. They were also told that the patient, being prone to having allergies, was likely to have that type of conjunctivitis. It was also explained to them that his allergic predisposition was familial, considering that Asthma, an allergic condition, was present in his family.

The eyelash within the right conjunctiva was removed using moist cotton-tipped bud, and his eyes were washed with sterile saline. He was placed on Antallerge (Antazoline hydrochloride 0.05%/ Tetrahydrozoline hydrochloride 0.04 g %) eye drops, with one drop to be instilled into each eye 6 hourly for 6 weeks. He was also given oral tablets of Loratadine 10 mg daily for 5 days because of his allergic predisposition. His mother was asked to inform his class teacher and school nurse about the condition and show them how to instill the eye drops in the patient's eyes at the appropriate time. He was to avoid dust, wool, and certain foods that were identified as allergens. The importance of regular hand washing was emphasized, noting that scratching his eyes with dirty hands could lead to the development of a secondary bacterial infection of the conjunctivae. He and his mother were advised to avoid instilling any medication or other substances into his eyes other than what had been prescribed, as well as to avoid ingesting drugs that were not prescribed, such as Phenergan. Furthermore, the patient was encouraged to continue schooling as his illness was not an infective condition. He was subsequently given a one-week appointment.

One-week follow-up:

The patient was seen a week later with his mother.

There was no eye swelling or discharge, and they were asked to continue instilling the eye medication. They were educated on the importance of good general and eye hygiene, which included washing their eyes with clean water whenever he felt a foreign body within his eyes rather than rubbing with his fingers. Thereafter, he was given a one-month appointment.

One-month follow-up:

When seen one month later, there was a complete resolution of his symptoms. Subsequently, he was discharged from follow-up.

Discussion:

A 9-year-old boy with a family history of atopy was diagnosed with Allergic conjunctivitis. His management involved medical treatment and health education on eye hygiene and avoidance of allergens. Allergic conjunctivitis is the inflammation of the conjunctiva as a result of a reaction to an allergen.[1] It constitutes one of the commonest eye diseases seen in many out-patient consultations all over the world and is estimated to affect between 20-40% of the population.[1-4]

The prevalence appears to be higher in younger age groups as was seen in the index patient who was a 9-year-old boy. In a study done among school children in Zaria, Nigeria, Abah et al. reported allergic conjunctivitis to be the most common ocular disorder among children with eye disorders.[5]

The disease presents with redness of the eyes, ocular itching, swelling of the eyelids, watery discharge from the eyes, photophobia, foreign body sensation, and pain in some cases.[1] The index patient presented with ocular itching, redness of the eyes, eyelid swelling, watery discharge, and foreign body sensation in his eyes. This led to the diagnosis of allergic conjunctivitis. Other forms of conjunctivitis exist and include bacterial conjunctivitis, viral conjunctivitis, gonococcal and chlamydial conjunctivitis.[2]

It was unlikely that this patient had bacterial conjunctivitis because, in bacterial conjunctivitis, the eye discharge is usually purulent, may affect only one eye and the patients usually have a history of a sinus or ear infection.[2,3] In viral conjunctivitis, the disease is highly contagious because it is spread by contact with infected eye secretions.[2,4] Contact with a person who had similar symptoms is a key feature in the etiology. Therefore, it is common among school children and other crowded populations because they have a great deal of contact with each other. This differential was excluded because of the patient's past medical history and family history of atopy.

Allergic conjunctivitis is a Type 1 hypersensitivity reaction. Type 1 hypersensitivity reaction is an allergic reaction provoked by re-exposure to a specific type of antigen called an allergen.

The antigen crosslinks preformed immunoglobulin E (IgE) on pre-sensitized mast cells, leading to degranulation and release of histamine and other inflammatory mediators.[6,7] Exposure may be through ingestion, inhalation, injection, or direct contact.[6,7]

The allergens may be aero-allergens or non-aeroallergens. They include pollen, fungal spores, fern spores, dust, air pollution, smoke, house mites, animal dander, cosmetics, contact lenses, sutures, eye drops, and prostheses following eye surgery.[7] Examples of Type 1 hypersensitivity reactions are anaphylaxis, food allergies, pollen allergies, and allergic rhinoconjunctivitis.[7]

Affected patients have a likely predisposition to atopy, which refers to a genetic tendency to develop allergic diseases. In this patient, there was a strong risk factor for allergy as it had been identified that he was allergic to dust, fomites, and some foods and had undergone similar symptoms twice within the previous year.

He also had a familial predisposition, as it was seen that his grandfather and other close relatives suffered from asthma. These factors significantly backed up the diagnosis.

The diagnosis is generally made by a thorough history and careful clinical observation. In this case, there was a detailed effort to establish a clear diagnosis and rule out other forms of conjunctivitis. Careful attention was also given to the past medical history, family, and social history to establish the patient's predisposition to atopy.

The disease can be treated with a variety of medications, including topical antihistamines, mast cell stabilizers, non-steroidal anti-inflammatory drugs, decongestants, artificial tears, and corticosteroids.[8,9] Surgery is also an option in rare cases of intractable keratoconjunctivitis.[8] Treatment of the index patient was achieved using a dual-acting topical eye preparation, which contained a decongestant and an antihistamine. The choice of these drugs was based on effectiveness, availability, and cost.

Steroids, though being the most effective drug in the treatment of allergic conjunctivitis, were avoided in this patient because of their severe side effects, which include ptosis, increased intraocular pressure, immune suppression, and secondary infection.[8, 9]

The primary behavioral modification for all types of allergic conjunctivitis is avoidance of the offending allergen.[10] In the management of this patient, he and his mother were educated on his illness; the allergens were identified, and he was advised to avoid them. He was also advised to maintain proper eye and hand hygiene by frequent handwashing.

Challenges in the management of this patient comprised inaccurate beliefs of the etiology of the disease by his caregivers, difficulty in the application of the topical eye drops over a long duration (6 weeks), the occurrence of the disease during an active school term, and the general difficulties of poor adherence encountered in the management of a pediatric patient. These challenges were overcome by proper health education of the child and his mother, as well as enlisting the help of the school nurse in the application of eye drops during school hours, following the correct dosage and timing.

Lessons Learned/recommendations:

Eye health education is necessary at the primary care level for children, adults, and caregivers. Family physicians should take the extra step in helping patients to identify possible allergens through proper health education.

References

1. Malu KN. Allergic conjunctivitis in Jos – Nigeria. Niger Med J 2014; 55: 166-70

2. Adenuga OO, Samuel OJ. Pattern of eye diseases in an air force hospital in Nigeria. Pak J Ophthalmol 2012; 28:144-8

3. Wade PD, Iwuora AN, Lopez L, Muhammad MA. Allergic conjunctivitis at sheikh zayed regional eye care center, Gambia. J Ophthalmic Vis Res 2012; 7:24-8.

4. Gomes PJ. Trends and prevalence of treatment of ocular allergy. Curr Opin Allergy Clin Immunol. 2014; 14(5): 451 - 456

5. Abah ER, Oladigbolu KK, Samaila E, Gani-Ikilama A. Ocular disorders in children in Zaria children's school. Niger J Clin Pract 2011; 14:473-6.

6. Matsuda A, Ebiharara N, Yokoi N, Kawasaki S, Inatomi T, et al. Functional role of thymic stromal

lymphopoietin in chronic allergic keratoconjunctivitis. Invest Ophtalmol Vis Sci 2010; 51: 151-5

7. Dimphna N, Ezikanyi GS, Nnamani CV. Aeroallergens in North Central Nigeria. Allergologia et Immunopathologia 2018; 46: 599-606

8. Davis S. Topical treatment options for allergic conjunctivitis. South African Family Practice. 2015; 57(4): 10 - 15

9. Bielory BP, Perez VL, Bielory L. Treatment of seasonal allergic conjunctivitis with ophthalmic corticosteroids: In search of the perfect ocular corticosteroids in the treatment of allergic conjunctivitis. Curr Opin Allergy Clin Immunol 2010; 10: 469-77

10. Choi H, Lee HB. Nonseasonal allergic conjunctivitis in the tropics: Experience in a tertiary institution. Ocul Immunol Inflamm 2008; 16(4):141-5

Chapter Two

External Hordeolum In A Make-Up Artist

A 24-year-old female make-up artist came to the clinic with pain and swelling on the right eyelid of four days' duration; and discharge from the right eye of a day's duration. She had been apparently well until four days before her clinic visit when she woke up feeling pain in her right upper eyelid.

On looking in the mirror, she noticed a slight swelling of the eyelid, which she thought would resolve as the day progressed. However, the swelling increased in size, and the pain continued. The day she came to the clinic, she noticed that pus discharged from the eye swelling in addition, there was itching of the right eyelid, tearing of the right eye, and dried particles on the eyelashes. She had no photophobia, and her vision was not affected.

A day before the onset of symptoms, she had forcefully pulled off her false eyelashes. She admitted that she frequently shared cosmetic eyepencils with her friends and also used cosmetic contact lenses. She had not recently changed her eye cosmetics to new formulations. Initially, she had sought treatment at a patent drug store where she was given eye drops that she applied for two days. She also applied a hot balm to the eye swelling as a remedy, but there was no relief rather, the symptoms became worse. So, she decided to visit the hospital for proper medical care. She felt that the condition was because she had forcefully removed her false eyelashes a day prior to the onset of the illness, and she was afraid that she would lose her sight. The illness had prevented her from leaving her house to attend to her personal concerns. She expected that her eye would be properly examined and treated,

She had no headache, sneezing, catarrh, itching of the throat, or cough. There was no history of asthma, diabetes, epilepsy, or hypertension. She had never had any surgical operations or blood transfusions. She was not on any routine drugs and was not allergic to any drugs or foods. The patient first had her menstruation at the age of eleven. Her menstrual flow lasted five days, while her cycle length was 28-30 days. There was no history of dysmenorrhea or menorrhagia. She was $P0^{+1}$. She terminated a pregnancy when she was 19 years old, and there had been no complications. She was sexually active and used barrier contraception occasionally.

She was the youngest child in a family of five children. Her parents and siblings were alive and well. She was a university graduate who was waiting to do the mandatory National Youth Service Corp program. Her source of finance was primarily from her parents, but she worked as a make-up artist occasionally, earning about N5,000 to

N10,000 per job. She lived in a rented two-bedroom apartment with her three friends. She was in an intimate relationship with a 32-year-old businessman and frequently indulged in both protected and unprotected sexual intercourse. She took alcohol (beer) occasionally and did not take tobacco in any form. Assessment of family APGAR was 10/10 and source of healthcare financing was out-of-pocket.

The examination revealed a young woman with a swollen upper right eyelid. She was not febrile, jaundiced, or dehydrated. She had a heart-shaped tattoo on her right shoulder. There was no peripheral lymphadenopathy or pedal oedema. An examination of the left eye showed that visual acuity was 6/6, the vision was preserved in all the fields, the cornea was transparent, the anterior chamber was of normal depth, the left pupil was bilaterally symmetrical with the right pupil, a normal red reflex was seen, and the retina was normal. In the right eye, visual acuity was 6/6, and vision was preserved in all fields of the right eye. A tender swelling, located externally, was seen on the medial aspect of the margin of the right upper eyelid. There was pus within the swelling with a purulent discharge on the eyelid. The conjunctiva was not injected. The right cornea was transparent, and the anterior chamber was of normal depth. A normal red reflex was elicited in the right eye, and the retina was normal.

She was conscious and well-oriented. There was no sign of meningeal irritation or cranial nerve deficit. Her motor and sensory systems were normal. Her pulse rate was 68 cycles per minute, regular with a full volume. Her blood pressure was 120/75 mmHg. The first and second heart sounds were heard. Her respiratory rate was 16 cycles per minute. She had equal chest expansion, and breath sounds were vesicular. Her abdomen was flat, soft, and moved with respiration. There was no tenderness elicited or organomegaly. Bowel sounds were normoactive.

A provisional diagnosis of External hordeolum was made. Differential diagnoses included chalazion, eyelid contact dermatitis, and peri-orbital cellulitis.

The diagnosis and management plan were carefully explained to the patient. She was reassured and told that the condition would not lead to blindness as it would be properly managed. Laboratory investigations included microscopy and culture of the eye discharge to know the implicating organism and affirm the diagnosis. A swab of the purulent discharge was obtained.

Following this, the patient's right eye was thoroughly washed with sterile injection water, and then, with the eyes closed, baby shampoo and gauze were used to clean the crusted discharge on the eyelashes. A warm compress was then applied to the right eye for some minutes.

She was told to repeat these procedures at home every six hours and was given oral tablets Diclofenac 75mg 12-

hourly for three days and broad-spectrum antibiotic tablets Amoxicillin/Clavulanate 625mg 12-hourly for five days.

She was counseled to avoid introducing foreign materials like false eyelashes and contact lenses into her eyes, as this was the likely cause of her illness. She was educated on the dangers of sharing personal items such as eye pencils, mascara, face towels, handkerchiefs, cosmetic brushes, and other cosmetics with her friends, as it was an easy way of contracting eye infections. Health education on good hygiene, regular hand washing, and daily facial cleansing to remove oils and dirt accumulated by cosmetics was imparted. Furthermore, she was warned against applying traditional eye medications or non-prescription eye drops from the patent drug store into her eyes.

The value of regular routine eye checks was emphasized. Since she had revealed that she regularly engaged in unprotected sex, the patient was counselled on safer sex practices which included abstinence, use of condoms, prevention of sexually transmitted infections through available vaccinations like the Hepatitis B vaccine, prompt testing for as well as treatment of sexually transmitted infections. Subsequently, she was given a three-day clinic appointment.

Three days follow-up:

When she was seen three days later, there was complete resolution of her symptoms. The result of the eye swab m/c/s showed the presence of Staphylococcus aureus sensitive to Ampicillin. Since she was responding to treatment with Amoxicillin/Clavulanate tablets, her medications were not changed, and she was encouraged to complete the medications. Thereafter, she was scheduled for a one-week appointment.

A definitive diagnosis of External hordeolum was made.

One-week later:

She did not have any complaints and had completed her medications. There was no swelling or pain in her eyes. Subsequently, the patient was discharged from follow-up.

Summary:

A 24-year-old make-up artist who was diagnosed with external hordeolum of the right eye. The condition was precipitated by the forceful removal of her false eyelashes. Also, she had a social history of indulging in risky sexual behavior. She was managed with medications, eyelid toileting as well as counselling on eye hygiene and safer sex practices.

Discussion:

A hordeolum, also known as a stye, is a painful inflammation of the eyelid margin caused by a bacterial infection.[1] It is one of the most common diseases of the eye seen in primary care however, incidence rates are largely unknown because the condition is not often reported.[2]

Although it tends to occur in younger people, there is no age, gender, or racial predilection.[2] The index patient was a young woman who presented with a painful swelling on the margin of her right upper eyelid.

Hordeolum can present with a lump on the top or bottom of the eyelid, localized swelling of the eyelid, pain, redness, itching, drooping of the eyelid, crusting of the eyelid margins, tearing, mucous discharge from the eye, light sensitivity and foreign body sensation.[2,3]

The patient presented with swelling on her eyelid, pain, purulent eye discharge, and crusting of the eyelid margin. These symptoms made the diagnosis appear straightforward; however, it was important to identify other eye conditions having similar presentations so as to clinically differentiate them. A chalazion presents with a swelling on the middle of the eyelid, tearing and redness of the conjunctiva.[4] However, the swelling is painless and tends to grow over time, unlike a hordeolum where the swelling is painful, and the onset is sudden. Periorbital cellulitis presents with swelling of the eyelid, but the swelling is more generalized and there may be additional systemic symptoms like fever.[4] This patient did not have other systemic symptoms.

In eyelid contact dermatitis, even though there would be a history of exposure to irritant agents such as eyeliners, eye makeup removers, eye shadows, and other facial cosmetics, the patient may have an additional history of allergy with symptoms like burning, stinging, or marked pruritus. Medical history may also indicate that the patient had changed cosmetic formulations thus giving rise to an allergic reaction. This patient did not have a history of allergy and had not recently changed her cosmetics.

The disease is usually caused by a bacterial infection of an oil gland in the eyelid, and the causative organism is *Staphylococcus aureus*.[3,5] There are currently no records of other causative organisms.

In the index patient, a microscopic culture of the purulent eye discharge revealed *S. aureus* as the causative organism, and this helped affirm the diagnosis.

The resulting inflammation can be internal, affecting the meibomian glands or it could be an external inflammation affecting the gland of Zeis.[5] In some cases, it could spread to other ocular tissues, resulting in periorbital cellulitis.[5] In this patient, the inflammation was external. Predisposing factors include lack of hygiene, poor nutrition, sleep deprivation, lack of water, and rubbing of the eyes.[6] In recent times, fashion trends among young ladies may contribute to the etiopathogenesis of hordeolum, which was the reason this case was reported. The use of cosmetic contact lenses, mascara, eye pencils, and artificial eyelashes, as well as its removal, could be a means of introducing bacteria into the eye and causing hordeolum.[7] In this patient, the likely predisposing factors were the forceful removal of false eyelashes and poor eye hygiene due to regular sharing of cosmetic tools; therefore, she was health educated on the dangers of introducing foreign materials into her eyes and cosmetic sharing.

In many cases, the lesions are self-limiting as they can drain spontaneously without the need for medical care.[8] However, treatment for this condition may be medical, surgical, or conservative.[8]

The application of warm compresses and eyelid toileting using baby shampoo and water are conservative treatments that can be used as an initial measure. Antibiotic eye ointment (such as Penicillin ointment), antibiotic eye drops (Chloramphenicol, erythromycin eye drops), and oral antibiotics can also be administered.[9] Surgical intervention like incision and drainage, may be used in cases where hordeolum fails to resolve after about a week of warm compresses.[9]

Other remedies that have been used in the management of hordeolum include acupuncture, autohemotherapy, digital massage, and home therapies like lid scrub and heated compresses.[9,10] In this patient, warm compresses were applied, and oral antibiotics were also administered in order to prevent possible pre-orbital cellulitis due to the presence of a considerable quantity of pus present within the eyelid.

Lessons learned/recommendations:

This case showed that the fashion trend of using artificial eyelashes by women had become a potential risk factor for eye infections. It is recommended that health education on eye care among ladies should incorporate either avoidance of these foreign materials on the eyes or hygienic application when they are used.

References

1. Sethuraman U, Kamat D. The red eye: evaluation and management. Clinical Pediatrics.2009; 48(6):588-600.
2. Lindsley K, Nichols JJ, Dickersin K. Interventions for acute internal hordeolum. Cochrane Database of Systematic Reviews 2013, Issue 4.
3. Panicharoen C, Hirunwiwatkul P. Current pattern treatment of hordeolum by ophthalmologists in Thailand. Journal of the Medical Association of Thailand 2011;94(6):721-4.
4. Lindsley K, Nichols JJ, Dickersin K. Non-surgical interventions for acute internal hordeolum. *Cochrane Database Syst Rev*. 2017; 1(1):CD007742.
5. Cheng K, Wang X, Guo M, Wieland LS, Shen X, Lao L. Acupuncture for acute hordeolum. Cochrane Database of Systematic Reviews 2014;4

6. Villines Z. Twelve causes and treatments of a swollen eyelid. *Medical News Today.* 2017, March 14. https://www.medicalnewstoday.com/articles/318219

7. Boyd K. What are chalazia and styes? 2016, September https://www.aao.org/eye-health/diseases/what-are-chalazia-styes

8. Uhumwangho OM, Kayoma DH. Current trends in treatment outcomes of orbital cellulitis in a tertiary hospital in Southern Nigeria. Niger J Surg. 2016; 22:107-10

9. Monsudi KF, Azonobi IR, Ayanniyi AA. Pattern of red eye in a tertiary eye clinic in Nigeria. Afr J Med Health Sci. 2015; 14:101-4

10. Oladigbolu KK, Abah ER, Chinda D, Anyebe EE. Pattern of eye diseases in a university health service clinic in northern Nigeria. Niger J Med 2012; 21:334-7.

Chapter Three

Recurrent Pelvic Inflammatory Disease In A 28-Year-Old Woman With Multiple Sexual Partners

Abnormal vaginal discharge of 6 months, abnormal vaginal bleeding of 2 months, and lower abdominal pain of one week in a 28-year-old female bank staffer.

The patient's symptoms began 6 months prior to her hospital visit when she noticed that she had a copious, creamy, and offensive vaginal discharge. Her menstrual periods had been irregular in the previous 2 months, with a sparse flow lasting 2-3 days as opposed to her regular flow of 5 days. She also observed that after her menstrual periods, she had abnormal vaginal bleeding, which could occur for about 1-2 days; this had happened many times.

About a week before her clinic visit, she developed lower abdominal pain that was of sudden onset, worse in the suprapubic region, continuous and sharp. It radiated to the lower back and was relieved with analgesics (Cataflam and Paracetamol). It was initially mild but gradually worsened until she was no longer responding to analgesics. There was a fever that was intermittent and low-grade. There was no history of recent termination of pregnancy, early morning vomiting, breast tenderness, or fainting attacks. The patient was sexually active and had a history of unprotected coitus with multiple sexual partners within the past 2 years. She also touched her vagina monthly. There was a history of similar symptoms within the past year for which she had been treated by a doctor. For her current symptoms, she had sought treatment from pharmacies, and alternative medicine shops and had been given drugs like Cataflam, Paracetamol, Doxycycline, Flagyl, Ciprofloxacin, Augmentin and herbal womb cleansers. When she did not have any improvement in the symptoms, she visited the hospital. The patient feared that due to the recurrent nature of her illness, she would become infertile. She assumed that her illness was due to inadequate treatment by the doctor who had treated her previously. The abdominal pain had prevented her from going to work, and she expected to be cured of the illness and her fertility preserved.

There was no urinary frequency, urgency, or change in color or odor of urine. There was no headache, vomiting, cough, chest pain, or difficulty in breathing. There was no history of hypertension, diabetes, asthma,, or epilepsy. There was no history of previous surgeries or blood transfusions.

Her first menstruation was at 12 years of age; she had a regular 28-day cycle with menstrual flow of 5 days. Her last menstrual period was 21 days before her clinic visit and lasted 3 days. For contraception, she used combined oral contraceptive pills and condoms occasionally. She was Para

0^{+2}, having undergone 2 terminations of pregnancy when she was 18 and 21 years, respectively. The procedures were done at private clinics, and gestational ages were between 8 and 12 weeks. There were no reported complications.

She was the first of 5 children, with two male and two female siblings. Her mother was a seamstress and lived in their hometown. Her father died when she was 16 years old. Assessment of family APGAR score was 7 out of 10 depicting a moderately dysfunctional family. She was a marketing officer at a commercial bank and earned a modest salary. She lived in a rented two-bedroom apartment with two younger siblings currently in the university, whose upkeep she was responsible for. Her sexual debut was at 17 years of age, and she was currently in sexual relationships with three different partners where she engaged in both protected and unprotected vaginal sexual intercourse. This had been going on for about two years.

On examination, the patient was ill-looking and febrile with a temperature of 38° C. She was neither pale nor dehydrated. She was anicteric and didn't have cyanosis. Her abdomen was flat, soft, and moved with respiration. There was tenderness in the hypogastrium and right and left iliac regions. The liver and spleen were not palpable, nor were her kidneys ballotable. Her bowel sounds were present and normoactive.

The pelvic examination showed normal external genitalia with no visible discharge or bleeding. There were no genital lesions and no protrusions from the vagina. Examination with a speculum showed copious mucopurulent and malodorous discharge in the vagina and posterior fornix. Her cervix was central with no abnormal lesions. There was a yellowish discharge from the cervical os, and the speculum was stained with malodorous yellowish discharge. A bimanual examination revealed that the uterus was anteverted and of normal size, mobile, and tender. There was adnexal tenderness, but the adnexa had no palpable masses. Cervical excitation tenderness was markedly positive, and the examining finger was stained with malodorous yellowish vaginal discharge.

Her pulse rate was 84 beats per minute, with a regular rhythm and normal volume. The blood pressure was 100/70mmHg. The patient's first and second heart sounds were heard. Her respiratory rate was 18 cycles per minute, and her chest moved with respiration. There was equal chest expansion. Her breath sounds were vesicular, and the chest was clinically clear. Examination of other systems did not reveal abnormalities.

A diagnosis of Pelvic Inflammatory Disease (PID) was made.

The diagnosis and management plan, which included a need for admission for administration of intravenous drugs, were explained to the patient, and she was admitted into the ward. The laboratory investigations that were requested included pregnancy test, complete blood count, urine analysis, endocervical swab (ECS) m/c/s, Chlamydia antibody test, HIV screening, and Hepatitis B/C screening. Abdomino-pelvic ultrasound scan was also requested.

The pregnancy test was negative, thus excluding pregnancy and ectopic pregnancy. She was commenced on intravenous Ceftriaxone 1g 12 hourly, intravenous Metronidazole 500mg 8 hourly, intravenous Gentamicin 80mg 8 hourly, and rectal Diclofenac 75mg 12 hourly, all for 48 hours.

First day of admission:

The patient was no longer having abdominal pain and had visibly improved. Her vital signs were within normal limits. The results of investigations showed that packed cell volume was 34%, erythrocyte sedimentation rate (ESR) was 20 mm/hr., and total white cell count was $10.6 \times 10^9/l$, with a differential count of 68% neutrophils, 31% lymphocytes, and eosinophil 1%.

Urine analysis displayed normal parameters. Hepatitis B surface antigen, Hepatitis C, and HIV screenings were non-reactive. Abdomino-pelvic ultrasound scan revealed ascitic fluid in the peritoneal cavity, increased vascularity, and thickening of the endometrium, with thickened fallopian tubes, thus suggesting pelvic inflammatory disease.

2nd – 3rd days of admission:

Following 48 hours of intravenous antibiotics, the patient was noted to have made a significant recovery. Intravenous antibiotics were continued for the following 24 hours thereafter. She had no new complaints, and her vital signs were normal.

Endocervical swab culture yielded Streptococcus agalactiae after 48hours' incubation which was sensitive to ceftriaxone (++), levofloxacin (+++), Augmentin (+), ciprofloxacin

(++), and erythromycin (+). The gram stain was positive for gram positive rods, gram negative rods, and gram-positive cocci. The chlamydial antibody test was positive for Chlamydia trachomatis antibodies. She was counselled on the possible causes and risk factors of her illness which included, in her case, multiple sexual partners, unprotected sex, and vaginal douching. This contrasted with her belief that she had been improperly treated when she had similar symptoms in the past. She was advised on safer sex, which involved either abstinence or adhering to one partner, and the correct and consistent use of condoms to prevent the recurrence of her illness, unplanned pregnancies leading to abortions, and sexually transmitted infections, including HIV and infertility in the long term.

She was also advised to stop vaginal douching as this could cause epithelial damage to the vagina, thereby increasing the risk of PID. Furthermore, she was counseled to abstain from sexual intercourse until the completion of her therapy and bring her sexual partners for treatment.

The patient acknowledged that though she had engaged in high-risk sexual behavior, it was for extra financial support since she was her widowed mother's major financial helper. The physician advised her to rather try to get employment for her siblings or even start small-scale businesses for them instead of putting her health and fertility at risk. Subsequently, she was discharged on the following drugs: Doxycycline tablets 100mg orally twice daily for 14 days, Metronidazole tablets 400mg orally thrice daily for 14 days, and Levofloxacin tablets 500mg daily for 7 days.

She was given Levofloxacin because her endocervical swab results reported the highest sensitivity to the drug; Metronidazole to treat anaerobes, and Doxycycline to treat chlamydial organisms, which had been identified with the Chlamydial antibody test. Intravenous Gentamicin and

Ceftriaxone were discontinued. Subsequently, she was given a one-week appointment.

One-week follow-up visit:

The patient was seen one week later and had recovered significantly. She was accompanied to the visit by her boyfriend, whom she had decided to settle down with, and he was given tablets of Levofloxacin 750 mg daily orally for 5 days, tablets of Doxycycline 100mg twice daily for 5 days, and tablets of Metronidazole 400mg 8-hourly for 5 days. She was advised to do a Pap smear and get immunized for Hepatitis B virus since she had never been immunized. She would receive three doses of the vaccine at 1st dose, 4 weeks after the first dose and 6 months after the first dose.

In the event whereby she had to travel out of the country in a month's time, she would take the second dose immediately after she returned, or she would take it at a health facility in the country that she traveled to. She was also asked to visit the clinic for one-month, three-month, and six-month visits to do endocervical swab tests. Regarding her family commitments, she was in the process of getting her brother's part-time employment at a departmental store to relieve her of some financial burden of their upkeep.

3-6 months follow-up:

In the ensuing tests, no abnormalities were detected. Further HIV screenings done at 3 months and 6 months were non-reactive. By her 6 months' visit, she had received 3 doses of Hepatitis B vaccine given at 1st dose, 4 weeks after the 1st dose and 6 months after the first dose. In all her visits, advice for safer sex was repeated. Her brothers had been gainfully employed, and she was in a relationship with one partner. She was eventually discharged from the outpatient clinic following her total recovery.

Summary:

A 28-year-old female banker with a history of vaginal discharge, bleeding, and abdominal pain and a social history of unprotected sexual intercourse with multiple sexual partners for financial gain. She was managed medically and with proper counseling on safer sex practices.

Discussion:

Pelvic inflammatory disease (PID) is a spectrum of inflammatory disorders of the upper female genital tracts, including any combination of endometritis, salpingitis, tubo-ovarian abscess, and pelvic peritonitis.[1,2] Risk factors for the development of PID include young age at sexual debut, previous PID history or sexually transmitted infection, new, multiple, or symptomatic sexual partners, use of non-barrier contraception, and vaginal douching.[3,4,5,7]. The index patient was a young, sexually active woman with multiple partners who regularly engaged in unprotected intercourse, and the risk factors included vaginal douching, previous history of PID, and unprotected sexual activity.

The clinical features of PID include fever, abnormal cervical or vaginal discharge, lower abdominal pain, and uterine, adnexal or cervical motion tenderness.[7] Atypical symptoms such as right upper quadrant pain from perihepatitis (Fitz-Hugh-Curtis syndrome) have been known to exist.[2] This patient presented with abnormal vaginal discharge, vaginal bleeding, and lower abdominal pain, which were typical symptoms of the disease. The etiological agents in most infections are *Chlamydia trachomatis* and *Neisseria gonorrhoea* even though organisms such as *Gardnerella vaginalis, Haemophilus influenza, Streptococcus agalactiae,* and enteric gram-negative rods have been implicated. [3-6] The organism isolated from the endocervical culture of the index patient was *S. agalactiae*. Chlamydial antibody test was also positive for Chlamydia trachomatis antibodies.

Complications of the disease include chronic pelvic pain, ectopic pregnancy, and infertility.[6, 7] It has been postulated that having this disease for as many as three times carries a 50% likelihood of a woman becoming infertile.[2] Infertility was a major concern for this patient as she feared that the recurrent nature of the disease would destroy her fertility. This issue was addressed by correct, effective treatment and extensive health education on safer sex practices known to be effective preventive measures against sexually transmitted infections and complications like infertility.

Social determinants of pelvic inflammatory disease were a key factor in this patient's illness experience. The recurrent nature of the disease was linked to multiple sexual contacts and the financial gain derived from them. Multiple sexual partners can be described as engaging in sexual activity with two or more people within a specific time period.[8]

Low socioeconomic status has been significantly associated with pelvic inflammatory disease.[9] This could be because young females from low socioeconomic backgrounds commonly engage in sex for money, favors, or material goods, thereby putting them at risk of contracting sexually transmitted diseases.[9] The patient was from a low socioeconomic background and was the main financial support for her widowed mother and younger siblings.

She engaged in risky sexual practices for financial gain since her salary was insufficient to handle her commitments. Effective counseling and behavioural interventions have been known to bring about positive change in at-risk females.[9,10] In this case, it was noted that the index patient, after being counselled, was able to develop new ways of changing her family's financial state while desisting from risky sexual behavior.

Lesson learned/recommendations:

Dysfunctional family environments due to financial incapacity can result in risky sexual behavior and health risks like pelvic inflammatory disease.

It is recommended that family physicians should create more awareness on PID prevention, which will include safer sex practices. Counseling and screening are needed for high-risk populations.

References

1. Centre for Disease Control and Prevention. Sexually transmitted diseases 2010 treatment guidelines. Morb Mortal Wkly Rep 2010; 59: 63-7

2. Gradison M. Pelvic inflammatory disease. Am Fam Physician. 2012; 85(8):791-796

3. Oseni TI, Odewale MA. Socioeconomic status of parents and the occurrence of pelvic inflammatory disease among undergraduates attending Irrua Specialist Teaching Hospital, Irrua, Edo State, Nigeria. Niger Postgrad Med J 2017; 24:114-20

4. Soper DE. Pelvic inflammatory disease. *Obstet Gynecol.* 2010; 116 (2):419–428.

5. Olowe OA, Alabi A, Akindele AA. Prevalence and pattern of bacterial isolates in cases of pelvic inflammatory disease patients at a tertiary hospital in Osogbo, Nigeria. Environ Res J 2012; 6:308-11

6. Arinze AU, Onyebuchi NV, Israel J. Genital chlamydia trachomatis infection among female undergraduate students in University of Port Harcourt, Nigeria. Niger Med J. 2014; 55:9-13

7. Hosenfeld CB, Workowski KA, Berman S, Zaidi A, Dyson J, Mosure D, et al. Repeat infection with chlamydia and gonorrhea among females: a systematic review of the literature. Sex Transm Dis. 2009; 36 (8):478–489.

8. Exavery A, Lutambi AN, Mubyazi GM, Kweka K, Mbaruku G, Masanja H. Multiple sexual partners and condom use, and condom use among 10-19 year olds in four districts in Tanzania. BMC Public Health. 2011; 11(1): 490

9. Ekpenyong CE, Etukumana EA. Ethnicity, family socioeconomic inequalities, and prevalence of vaginal douching among college students: the implications for health. J Am Coll Health. 2013; 61: 222-30

10. Trent M, Chung SE, Burke M, Walker A, Ellen JM. Results of a randomized controlled trial of a brief behavioural intervention for pelvic inflammatory disease in adolescents. J Pediatr Adolesc Gynecol. 2010;23(2):96–101

Chapter Four

Septic Abortion In A High School Student

A 17-year-old female high school student presented with a fever of 3 days, lower abdominal pain, vaginal bleeding, and vaginal discharge of 1 week. She was apparently well until a week prior to the presentation when she developed lower abdominal pain. It was gradual in onset, continuous, radiated to the back and had no relieving or aggravating factors. There was associated nausea and dizziness. There was no history of ingestion of any substances or drugs prior to the onset of abdominal pain. She also had vaginal bleeding, and her blood was dark-red, malodorous and contained clots. The bleeding occurred intermittently, and when she was not bleeding, she observed a thick, copious, yellow, malodorous vaginal discharge. The fever occurred three days before her hospital admission and was of sudden onset, high-grade, continuous and associated with chills and rigor. She had two episodes of vomiting and vomitus, which contained fluid, and ingested food. A week prior to her visit, she had had an induced abortion for an eight-week-old pregnancy. The procedure involved instrumentation and was done by an untrained drug store attendant. Her immediate condition afterward was reported as uneventful, and she was not given any post-procedure medications.

At the onset of her symptoms, she drank palm oil in a bid to treat herself. Her mother gave her analgesics and an anti-malarial drug, thinking she had malaria, but when symptoms continued unabated, and her mother discovered that she had recently had an abortion, she took her to the emergency unit of the hospital. The patient feared that she would die from her illness, and she had the idea that she had eaten a poisonous substance. The illness had robbed her of school days, and she expected that her stomach would be pumped to remove any poison.

Her past medical and surgical history showed that she had no history of hypertension, diabetes, asthma or sickle cell disease. There was also no history of previous surgery or blood transfusion. Her obstetric and gynaecological history showed that the patient was a $P0^{+1}$ female. Her first menstruation occurred when she was 11 years old; the duration of her menstrual flow was 5 days, and her cycle length was regular at 28 – 30 days. There was a history of dysmenorrhea and the presence of blood clots within her menstrual flow. She had no history of contraceptive use.

Her family and social history showed that she was the second child in a family of 3 children, two females and one male. She was a senior student in a government secondary school. Both parents were alive; her mother was a teacher at a government primary school, while her father was a health inspector for the local government. Her father was a clergy in their local church. She was a non-smoker and did not drink alcohol. She became sexually active at the age of 16 and had been in two relationships from the onset of sexual activity. She was currently in a relationship with a fellow student and regularly had unprotected sexual intercourse. The assessment of family APGAR was 5/10 depicting a moderately dysfunctional family.

The physical examination showed the patient was acutely ill-looking, febrile with a temperature of 39.2^0C, pale, and dehydrated. She was neither icteric nor cyanosed and did not have significant peripheral lymphadenopathy or pedal oedema. Her pulse rate was 104 beats per minute with a regular rhythm and low volume. Her blood pressure was 90/60 mmHg; the apex beat was at the fifth left intercostal space along the mid-clavicular line. The first and second heart sounds were heard. Her respiratory rate was 20 cycles per minute. There was equal air entry on both lung fields, and breath sounds were vesicular. Her abdomen was flat and moved with respiration and some guarding. There was suprapubic tenderness but no enlarged organs.

In the pelvic examination, there was a malodorous mucopurulent discharge at the vulva. Examination with a speculum revealed a closed cervical os. There was mild bleeding and clots within the cervix. Adnexal tenderness and cervical excitation tenderness were present.

A diagnosis of Septic incomplete abortion was made.

Management:

The patient was managed as an emergency and immediately admitted to the Gynecological ward. Using a wide-bore cannula, she was given intravenous fluids. She was given a liter of Normal Saline over 30 minutes and subsequently 1 liter 4-hourly for 24 hours. She was catheterized, and a urine bag was attached to monitor urine output. The patient was further given intravenous

Ceftriaxone 1 gram 12 hourly, intravenous Metronidazole 500 mg 8 hourly, intravenous Gentamicin 80mg 8 hourly and intramuscular Diclofenac 75 mg 12 hourly, all for 48 hours.

The laboratory investigations that were done included pregnancy test, complete blood count, urinalysis, electrolyte, urea and creatinine assay, endocervical swab, HIV screening, Hepatitis screening, and VDRL test. The results obtained revealed a negative pregnancy test and protein +++ in the urine. The complete blood count results showed hemoglobin was 9.8gm/dl, white cell count 11.2×10^9/l with a differential count of 85% neutrophils, 14% lymphocytes and 1% eosinophils. HIV, Hepatitis B/C, and VDRL screenings were all negative. The electrolytes assay showed serum urea was 70 mmol/l, Na^+ 135 mmol/l, K^+ 111 mmol/l, Cl^- 96 mmol/l and HCO_3 22 mmol/l. Endocervical swab culture yielded chlamydial organisms on gram stain. A pelvic ultrasound scan, which was done, showed a bulky uterus having an irregular outline and some products of conception within the endometrial cavity.

A manual vacuum aspiration (MVA) was done for the patient. About 30 ml of retained products of conception and blood clots were obtained. There was no active bleeding at the end of the procedure. The specimen obtained from this procedure was sent for histopathological analysis. Her immediate condition after the procedure was stable, with vital signs of the pulse rate of 86 beats per minute, blood pressure 100/70mmHg, and temperature of 38.4 ^{0}C. Hydration was maintained using intravenous 5% Dextrose Saline solution 1 liter 8 hourly.

First day of admission:

On her first day of admission, she complained of mild abdominal pain and weakness. Her temperature was 38^0 C, pulse rate 80 beats per minute, blood pressure 110/80mmHg, and respiratory rate 18 cycles per minute.

Urine output over 24 hours was 320 ml. Drug administration and observation of the patient were continued thereafter.

2nd - 5th days of admission:

With constant drug administration, the patient made a visible recovery. Intravenous medications were discontinued after 48 hours on admission, and she was commenced on Cefuroxime tablets 750 mg twice daily for 10 days, Metronidazole tablets 400mg three times daily for 10 days, Diclofenac tablets 75 mg twice daily for 3 days, and iron syrup 10 ml twice daily for 14 days, all orally.

She was advised to get immunized for the Hepatitis B virus and counselled on safer sex practices, which included abstinence, avoidance of multiple sexual partners, and barrier contraception. Regarding contraception, she was educated on the importance of contraception and the various methods but was firmly advised that abstinence from pre-marital sex remained her best option.

The consequences of premarital sex were explained to her, and this explanation was backed up by the recent illness which she was recovering from. Abstinence would ensure that she avoided issues of unwanted pregnancy, unsafe abortions, sexually transmitted infections, and HIV/AIDS. Negative peer group influence was discussed, and the patient was encouraged to focus on her academics and extra-curricular activities such as sports, music, and church youth fellowships.

She was discharged after five days and given a follow-up appointment in one week.

First follow-up visit:

The patient attended her first follow-up visit a week later with her mother. She had no new complaints. Her mother stated how the entire illness episode had greatly stressed her and how she had kept it a secret from the patient's father, as he would publicly disown her if he ever knew about being a clergy in their church. She was, however, advised about the benefits of disclosure, being gently informed that both parents had a role to play in the health and welfare of the patient. A one-month clinic appointment was given.

Second follow-up visit:

At this visit, the patient had no complaints. She had completed all her medications. She had commenced active preparation for her senior secondary school certificate and university-entry examinations, which were due in a few months. Regarding her social life, she had discontinued her relationship with her boyfriend and was determined to avoid premarital sex.

She affirmed that she no longer kept company with peers who were involved in sexual relationships but was now more involved in church activities. Her mother was commended for the moral support she gave to her and encouraged to be even more vigilant in monitoring her progress.

Summary:

A 17-year-old girl was seen at the emergency room with vaginal discharge and bleeding after an induced abortion that became septic which was done by an untrained drug store attendant. Her mother's fear was possible family disintegration due to her father's strong negative views on premarital sex, unwanted pregnancy and contraception. Her management included manual vacuum aspiration and counselling on safer sex practices with an emphasis on abstinence.

Discussion:

Abortion has been defined as the expulsion or extraction from the mother of an embryo or fetus weighing 500 grams or less when it is not capable of independent survival.[1,2] The expulsion can be spontaneous, without any external manipulation, or induced either by medical, surgical, or other unorthodox means.[3] Abortion is usually complete when all products of conception have been expelled and incomplete when there are remnants of the products of conception.[1,2] A septic abortion is an infection of the placenta and fetus, or products of conception, of a pre-viable pregnancy.[3]

The index patient had an induced abortion of an eight-week old pregnancy and presented with symptoms and signs in keeping with septic incomplete abortion.

In developing nations, septic abortion remains a primary cause of maternal mortality,[4] quite unlike in developed nations where statistics are very low.[5] The World Health Organization reports that about 68,000 women in developing countries die each year from the complications of unsafe abortions.[4] In Nigeria, the official statistics may not be fully available because induced abortion is illegal in the country, and its practice is usually clandestine.[6,7] Septic abortions could occur as a result of unsafe techniques by individuals without the necessary skills and in an environment that does not conform to minimum medical standards or both.[6,7] This patient had an induced abortion performed by a drug store attendant who was a non-professional, and in a non-medical facility under septic conditions. The deficiency of requisite skills resulted in the retention of products of conception and subsequent pelvic infection. Complications of septic abortion include infertility, toxic shock, and death.[1-3]

Teenage pregnancy has further fueled the problem of septic abortion as it has been found that 14% of unsafe abortions in low and middle-income countries occur among teenagers aged 15-19 years.[9] Teenage pregnancy is a pregnancy that occurs between the ages of thirteen to nineteen years.[9]

At this age, most females are inexperienced and therefore physically, emotionally, financially and psychologically unfit to handle the responsibility of pregnancy.[9] Teenagers tend to conceal details of their activities from parents and guardians who would have a moderating influence on them but instead rely on peers for advice and usually end up in clandestine places for unsafe abortions.[9] Predisposing factors for teenage pregnancy include peer pressure, media influence, poverty, drug addiction, alcoholism, child neglect, sexual abuse, child marriage, poor knowledge, and poor access to contraception.[9] Where teenage pregnancy occurs, it presumes an early sexual debut by a female, and this has its own consequences like sexually transmitted infections, HIV/AIDS, cervical cancer, unwanted pregnancy, early marriage, poor academic performance and an increase in school dropout rates.[6,9] The index patient was a teenager who had an early sexual debut at 16 years. With no knowledge of contraception or the demands of pregnancy, she kept this issue from her parents and rather chose to have an unsafe abortion, which led to serious consequences.

Socio-cultural, religious, and individual factors have been known to influence the issue of abortions in many climes.[6-8] In Western countries, abortion has been widely accepted due to its legalization in those countries.[5] Access to contraceptive services has also been found to be invaluable in preventing unwanted pregnancies, thus reducing the risks of septic abortion in these countries.[9,10] However, in many parts of Africa including Nigeria, abortion is unacceptable as many people due to religious beliefs, sociocultural traditions and legal prohibition consider it murder.[6,7] Thus females who undergo abortions face intense stigmatization.[7]

Abortions have been known to cause family dysfunction and breakdown.[7] The patient and her mother, fearing a family breakdown, concealed the act from her father, who was a church leader. This action thus reflected a dysfunctional family unit because the ideal solution should have been for both parents to work together in helping the patient's social issues. The family APGAR is an important tool for the assessment of family functionality and was used in this patient's management.

Lessons Learned/Recommendations:

In secondary schools, youth groups, and adolescent clinics, teenagers should be made to understand the dangers of early sexual debut and unwanted pregnancy. There should be increased access to contraceptive services, which is the least expensive and most important preventive measure of septic abortion.

References

1. Stubblefield PG, Averbach SH, Grimes DA. Septic abortion: prevention and management. Glob. Libr. Women's med. 2012; vol. 6: chap. 118

2. Lim LM, Singh K. Termination of pregnancy and unsafe abortion. Best Pract Res Clin Obstet Gynaecol. 2014; Aug 28(6): 859-69

3. Eschenback, D. Treating Spontaneous and Induced Septic Abortions. Obstet Gynecol. 2015; 125:1042-1048.

4. Kassebaum N, Bertozzi-Villa A, Coggeshall M, et al. Global, regional, and national levels and causes of maternal mortality during 1990-2013: a systematic analysis for the global burden of disease study 2013. *Lancet.* 2014; 384:980-1004.

5. Pazol K, Creanga AA, Burley KD, Jamieson DJ. Abortion surveillance – United States, 2011. MMWR Surveill Summ. 2014 Nov 28. 63 Suppl 11: 1-41

6. Bankole A, Adewole IF, Hussain R, Awolude O, Singh S, Akinyemi JO. The incidence of abortion in Nigeria. Int Perspect Sex Reprod Health. 2015; 41(4):170–181. doi:10.1363/4117015

7. Emechebe CI, Njoku CO, Udofia UM, Ukaga JT. Complications of induced abortion: contribution to maternal mortality in a tertiary center of a low-resource setting. Saudi J Health Sci 2016; 5:34-8

8. Alabi OT, Oni IO. Teenage pregnancy in Nigeria: causes, effects and control. International Journal of Academic Research in Business and Social Sciences. 2017; 7:2

9. Owolabi OO, Biddlecom A, Whitehead HS. Health system's capacity to provide post-abortion care. The Lancet Global Health.2019; 7:1. doi:10.1016/S2214-109X(18)30404-2

10. Adinma JIB, Ikeako L, Adinma ED, Ezeama CO, & Ugboaja JO. Awareness and practice of post abortion

care services among health care professionals in southeastern Nigeria. The Southeast Asian J of Tropical Medicine and Public Health. 2010; 41:3. pp 696-704.

Chapter Five

Malaria In Pregnancy

A 35-year-old pregnant female teacher presented to the hospital with a fever and headache of 5 days' duration. The patient was a pregnant woman at 26 weeks gestational age who was apparently well until five days before presentation when she developed a fever which was high-grade, intermittent and associated with chills and rigors. She had a headache, which was generalized, throbbing in nature and persistent. Both symptoms were relieved temporarily by ingestion of Paracetamol.

A day before the presentation, she had four episodes of vomiting, which occurred immediately after every meal. Vomitus was bilious and contained recently ingested food. She had poor appetite, a bitter taste in the mouth, an inability to retain meals, generalized body pain, and weakness. There was no cough, chest pain, difficulty in breathing, yellowness of the eyes, abdominal pain, genital bleeding or discharge, change in bowel habits, or urinary symptoms.

At the onset of these symptoms, she had visited a private clinic where she was given Fansidar, an antimalarial drug, and Paracetamol, but she took only Paracetamol, refusing to take Fansidar because she thought that antimalarial drugs could kill the baby.

She had been told by friends and co-workers that pregnancy usually mimicked malaria symptoms. She even delayed booking at the antenatal clinic for antenatal care because she did not want to be given any drugs that would jeopardize her pregnancy, choosing only to take iron and folic acid tablets. However, due to the persistent vomiting, inability to retain meals, and increasing general weakness, she was brought to the hospital by her husband. She feared that treatment with drugs would harm her baby. She felt that her symptoms were due to pregnancy, being that this was her first confinement. The illness had prevented her from going to work. She expected that any treatment given to her would not harm her baby because this was a precious pregnancy.

Her past medical and surgical history showed she had no history of hypertension, diabetes, asthma, epilepsy, or sickle cell disease. There was a history of previous blood transfusions. She was taking folic acid and iron tablets, which were self-medicated.

There was no known allergy to any drugs and no known side effects to any drugs. Her obstetric and gynecological history showed she was primigravid. Her menarche was at 14 years of age, her menstrual cycle was between 30-45 days, and her menstrual flow was 3-4 days. She had never used any form of contraception. She had no history of terminations of pregnancy. The patient had suffered from primary infertility for six years after marriage. There was a history of galactorrhea that was treated with Bromocriptine. She had also done a myomectomy two years before the current visit and received two units of blood with no complications.

She was the second child in a family of five children. Only her mother was alive. She was a secondary school teacher and had been married for six years to a 39-year-old engineer with the State civil service. They lived in a rented two-bedroom apartment that had mosquito nets on the windows that were not insecticide-treated. She neither drank alcohol nor took tobacco in any form. The family was at the beginner's stage of Evelyn Duvall's model. The family APGAR score assessment was 8/10, showing a functional family. The source of healthcare financing was out-of-pocket.

The general physical examination showed the patient was acutely ill-looking, febrile with a temperature of 39.4°C, and mildly dehydrated. She was not pale, icteric, or cyanosed. There was no pedal oedema and no significant peripheral lymphadenopathy. Her pulse rate was 106 beats per minute. The pulse had a regular rhythm and full volume. Her blood pressure was 100/70 mmHg, and only the first and second heart sounds were heard. Her respiratory rate was 20 cycles per minute. She had equal chest expansion, resonant percussion notes, and vesicular breath sounds. In the abdominal examination, her abdomen was gravid, soft, and moved with respiration. There was no area of tenderness and no palpable organ enlargement. The symphysial-fundal height was 25 cm, which was compatible with her gestational age. Fetal heart sounds were heard, and fetal movement was felt.

A diagnosis of Malaria in pregnancy was made.

Management:

The diagnosis with management plan was explained to the patient including the need for admission. She was assured that the medications given to her would not harm her baby but would prevent complications arising from the illness. Following this, she was admitted into the Antenatal ward. Laboratory investigations that were done included complete blood count, urine analysis, and blood film for malaria parasites. The results revealed a hemoglobin value of 10 g/dl, packed cell volume of 30%, and white cell count of 5.6×10^9 with differentials of 1% eosinophil, 55% neutrophils, and 44% lymphocytes. The blood film for malaria parasites showed ring forms of Plasmodium falciparum, and urine analysis showed normal parameters.

First day of admission:

She was given intravenous 5% Dextrose saline infusion one liter 8-hourly at 30 drops per minute for 24 hours, intramuscular Paracetamol 600mg stat dose to be followed orally with tablets Paracetamol 1000 mg 8-hourly for 3 days, intramuscular Promethazine 25 mg stat dose, and intramuscular Paluther (β-arteether) 150 mg daily for 3 days. Her vital signs were monitored six-hourly.

The second day of admission:

When seen, she complained of weakness. Her body temperature had dropped to 37.5°C; there had been no episode of vomiting, and fetal heart sounds were normal. Her medications were continued, and she was encouraged to eat.

3rd day of admission:

She had no complaints. A repeat blood smear for malaria parasites did not show any parasites. She was health-educated on malaria, the route of infection, complications, and prevention, being counseled on the importance of using insecticide-treated nets for the prevention of malaria. The role of antenatal care in the achievement of an optimal pregnancy outcome was emphasized and she was assured that the routine drugs prescribed during antenatal visits were safe for both mother and baby, with positive effects of improving immunity and preventing diseases. The patient was told to discard her wrong perspectives of malaria treatment during pregnancy and advised on good nutrition and adequate rest. She was given oral tablets of Lonart (artemether/lumefantrine) 80mg/480mg twice daily for 3 days, Fesolate 200 mg three times daily, and one tablet of Folic Acid (0.4mg or 400mcg) daily for one month. She was also booked for antenatal care, discharged, and given a 1-week appointment.

One-week follow-up:

The patient was seen at the antenatal clinic on her scheduled date. She did not have any complaints, and her general physical condition was stable. Thereafter, she was asked to continue with her routine antenatal visits until delivery.

This patient eventually gave birth at 40 weeks to a female child weighing 3.4kg through spontaneous vaginal delivery. The child cried at birth and had no reported anomalies.

Summary:

A pregnant 35-year-old secondary school teacher at 26-weeks' gestation was diagnosed with malaria, which was severe enough to require hospital admission. The patient's refusal to accept drug treatment due to her inaccurate perspective of the disease contributed to the severity of her illness. She was treated with parenteral medication and health education.

Discussion:

Malaria, an infection transmitted by mosquitoes, is the most devastating parasitic disease globally.[1] It affects between 350 – 500 million people annually and accounts for 1 – 3 million deaths per year.[1,2] It has a high impact on maternal health to the extent that of approximately 125.2 million women who become pregnant in malaria-endemic regions annually, 24 million are affected by the infection.[2] Pregnant women are highly susceptible because of the predilection of the parasites to sequester in the placenta.[3] The causative agent of malaria is Plasmodium species, which could be *P. falciparum, P. vivax, P. ovale, P. malariae* and *P. knowlesi*. The index patient was a pregnant woman diagnosed with Malaria.

The clinical features of malaria include the classic triad of fever, chills, and sweating, headache, musculoskeletal pain, asthenia, vomiting, and diarrhea.[1,4] In severe cases, it might present with an altered level of consciousness, convulsion, coluria (dark urine and presence of blood or haemoglobin in urine), jaundice, spontaneous bleedings, persistent vomiting, persistent diarrhoea, hyperpyrexia or hypothermia and severe dehydration.[4] In the index patient, the clinical features found were fever, headache, vomiting, musculoskeletal pain and asthenia.

The diagnosis can be through microscopy of stained blood smears, polymerase chain reaction (PCR), and placental histology.[3] Point-of-care rapid diagnostic tests (RDT) can also be used in diagnosis. Microscopy of blood smears remains the most widely used method for diagnosing malaria. The diagnosis of malaria in this patient was done using microscopy of blood smear.

The World Health Organization (WHO) recommends a three-pronged strategy for the control of malaria in pregnancy.[3,4]

This includes case management (prompt treatment with highly effective drugs), use of insecticide-treated nets (ITNs) as well as intermittent preventive treatment (IPTp), which is the administration of a full treatment course of an effective antimalarial (Sulphadoxine-pyrimethamine) at regular antenatal visits, usually a month apart.[4,5]

Based on the recommendation, women in their second or third trimesters with uncomplicated *P.falciparum* malaria are treated with artemisinin-based combination therapy.

This patient was treated with the artemether/lumefantrine combination due to its safety and efficacy profile.

Globally, there have been barriers faced in the management of malaria in pregnancy, which has made the disease one of the most challenging infectious diseases to eradicate.[6,7] These barriers are found at different levels, such as policy and guidance, healthcare provider performance, health system issues, and women's perspectives.[7,8]

Wrong perspectives, local cultural norms, household commitments, and traditional beliefs all constitute barriers from the women's perspective.[8] A study done among pregnant women in Mozambique indicated that many pregnant women do not perceive malaria as dangerous for the pregnancy and fetus, even though malaria is a well-known health problem in pregnancy.[10] An important deterrent to the use of antimalarial drugs is the fear that the drugs could cause harm to the unborn fetus and even lead to abortion.[9,11] In many cases, these beliefs are so firmly entrenched that they greatly impede the smooth delivery of healthcare services to women. This was evident in the index patient who, though well-educated at a tertiary institution, refused to take drugs prescribed by a doctor due to an inaccurate perception of her illness and poor information.

Lessons learned/Recommendations:

Inaccurate perspectives, cultural norms, and traditional beliefs tend to make malaria in pregnancy, a high-risk condition, appear trivial thus resulting in morbidity and mortality. It is recommended that family physicians must properly inform women attending antenatal clinics about the healthcare practices that would be given to them and directly address certain beliefs that could obstruct the effective treatment of malaria in pregnancy.

References

1. Piñeros JG, Tobon-Castaño A, Alvarez G, Portilla C, Blair S. Maternal clinical findings in malaria in pregnancy in a region of Northwestern Colombia. *Am J Trop Med Hyg.* 2013;89 (3):520–526.

2. Dellicour S, Tatem AJ, Guerra CA, Snow RW, ter Kuile FO. Quantifying the number of pregnancies at risk of malaria in 2007: A demographic study. PLoS Med. 2010; 7:1000221

3. Rogerson SJ. Management of malaria in pregnancy. *Indian J Med Res.* 2017;146 (3):328–333.

4. Guidelines for the Treatment of Malaria. 3rd edition. Geneva: World Health Organization; 2015. Available at https://www.ncbi.nlm.nih.gov/books/NBK294440.

5. Aguzie ION, Ivoke N, Onyishi GC, Okoye IC. Antenatal practices ineffective at prevention of plasmodium falciparum malaria during pregnancy in a

sub-Saharan Africa Region, Nigeria. *Trop Med Infect Dis.* 2017; 2(2):15.

6. Maung TM, Tripathy JP, Oo T, Oo MS, Soe TN, Thi A et al. Household ownership and utilization of insecticide-treated nets under the regional artemisinin resistance initiative in Myanmar. *Trop Med Health.* 2018; 46:27.

7. Ivoke N, Ivoke ON, Okereke NC, Eyo JE. *Plasmodium* malaria parasitaemia among pregnant women attending clinics in a Guinea-Savannah zone, Southern Ebonyi State, Nigeria. Int. J. Sc. Eng. Res. 2013; 4:1876–1883

8. Ofori MF, Ansah E, Agyepong I, Ofori-Adjei D, Hviid L, Akanmori BD. Pregnancy-associated malaria in a rural community of Ghana. Ghana Med J. 2009; 43:13–18.

9. Boene H, González R, Valá A, Rupérez M, Velasco C, Machevo S, et al. Perceptions of malaria in pregnancy

and acceptability of preventive interventions among Mozambican pregnant women: implications for the effectiveness of malaria control in pregnancy. PLoS ONE. 2014; 9(2): e86038.

10. Pell C, Straus L, Andrew EV, Menaca A, Pool R. Social and cultural factors affecting uptake of interventions for malaria in pregnancy in Africa: a systematic review of the qualitative research. PLoS One. 2011; 6(7)

Chapter Six

Retained Placenta In A 31-Year-Old Woman

A 31-year-old seamstress presented to the hospital with an inability to deliver the placenta about 1 hour after delivery. She was a pregnant woman at 41-week gestational age who went into spontaneous labor a day before the presentation. She had been taken to a maternity home owned by the local church she attended, where she had a spontaneous vaginal delivery of a live male infant that weighed 3.5kg. Following delivery, all attempts to deliver the placenta failed.

She was administered an Oxytocin injection intramuscularly, and bleeding was minimal. There was no history of weakness, dizziness, or fainting attacks. There was no fever, vomiting, leg swelling or convulsions. When all efforts to deliver the placenta by the birth attendant proved abortive, she was taken to the general hospital. The patient was afraid that she would die from this condition and regretted that she had not gone to deliver her baby at the hospital. She had the idea that the whole incident was a spiritual attack. She expected that the doctor would salvage the situation and she would be alive to care for her young children.

For the index pregnancy, she had booked for antenatal care at the General Hospital at a gestational age of 18 weeks. She kept all her antenatal appointments and received two doses of tetanus toxoid vaccine. The pregnancy was uneventful. She chose to deliver at the maternity home because it was affiliated with her church, and she wanted spiritual covering during childbirth. Her past medical and surgical history indicated there was no history of hypertension, diabetes mellitus, sickle cell anaemia, asthma, or epilepsy. There was no history of previous transfusions.

The patient was a $P4^{+2}$ (2 alive) lady. She had a history of termination of a confirmed 12-week pregnancy at a private clinic, which occurred 9 years prior to this hospital visit. There were no post-abortion complications. In her second pregnancy, she suffered a spontaneous miscarriage after about 10 weeks' gestation. An evacuation was done at the hospital. Subsequently, she had a normal pregnancy, which was booked and carried out to term. Labor was uneventful, and she had a spontaneous vaginal delivery of a live female infant, which weighed 3.3 kg. She delivered at a maternity home owned by her church. The child was alive and well. Her menarche occurred at 11 years of age. She had a menstrual cycle of 22-26 days with 4 days of menstrual flow. She used condoms occasionally as a method of contraception.

The patient was the third child in a family of 5 children, 2 females and three males. She was a seamstress married to a 37-year-old electrician. She took alcoholic beverages occasionally but did not take tobacco in any form. The family was at the school-age children's stage, according to Evelyn Duvall's staging. Assessment of family APGAR was 10/10, showing a functional family. The source of healthcare finance was out-of-pocket.

A physical examination revealed an anxious-looking woman who was not febrile, pale, icteric, cyanosed, or dehydrated. There was no pedal oedema. Her pulse rate was 90 beats per minute. Pulse had a regular rhythm and full volume. Her blood pressure was 120/80 mmHg, and she had normal heart sounds. Her respiratory rate was 18 cycles per minute, and her chest was clinically clear. Her abdomen showed a 16 week size uterus. The abdomen was firm and moved with respiration. There was suprapubic tenderness. There was no palpable enlargement of the liver or spleen. Her kidneys were not balloted. Vaginal examination revealed the vulva was blood-stained and had a clamped umbilical cord of about 15 cm in length extending from the vagina. The cervix was 100% effaced, and the cervical os was 6 cm dilated. There was no active bleeding.

A diagnosis of Retained placenta was made.

Management:

The diagnosis and management plan were quickly explained to the patient and her husband. She was booked for manual removal of the placenta after due counseling, and informed consent was obtained from her. Intravenous access was established using a wide-bore cannula (18G), and she was given 1liter of 5% Dextrose Saline containing 40 IU Oxytocin to run for an hour. Controlled cord traction was then attempted without success. She was catheterized, and about 120 ml of clear urine was drained from the bladder. An urgent packed cell volume was done and showed a value of 31%. Two units of blood were grouped and cross-matched. She was administered 1 gram of Ceftriaxone and 500 milligrams of Metronidazole, both intravenously.

In the theatre, the patient was placed in the lithotomy position. The procedure of manual removal of the placenta was done under an aseptic protocol, with the medical personnel being properly scrubbed, draped, and gloved. A surgical tray had been prepared with the necessary equipment. For premedication, she was given IV Atropine at 0.01mg/kg (0.6mg) and IV Diazepam at 0.3mg/kg. General anesthesia was achieved through total intravenous anesthesia (TIVA) using IV Ketamine 2mg/kg. Her external genitalia, abdomen, and thighs were cleaned with Chlorhexidine solution and draped. Following this, a pelvic examination was done on her. The findings were an intact vulva, vagina, and cervix, an umbilical cord of about 15 cm in length protruding from the vagina, cervical os dilatation of 6cm, and a normal uterine cavity with the placenta adherent to the anterior fundal region. The left hand was first placed on the abdomen to keep the uterus steady. With the fingers held closely together, the right hand was inserted into the vagina; the cervical os was identified, and through it, the uterine cavity was entered using the cord as a guide. The plane on the placental insertion in the uterine cavity was identified, and the placenta was gently sheared off from the uterine wall, starting from its lower pole. Following the complete separation of the placenta, 10 international units (IU) of Oxytocin were administered intravenously, and the placenta was then grasped with the hand and gently pulled out.

The placenta was inspected, and all the lobes were complete. The genital tract was also inspected and found to be intact. The uterus was well contracted, and there was no further bleeding following the removal of the placenta. The estimated blood loss was about 250 ml. The patient was administered 20 IU of Oxytocin in 500ml of 5% Dextrose Saline infusion to run for 4 hours. Blood was not transfused, and her immediate condition after the procedure was satisfactory.

The post-procedure medications that were given to the patient included intramuscular Pentazocine 30 mg stat, then tablets Diclofenac 50 mg 12 hourly orally for 5 days, tablets Cefuroxime 500 mg 12 hourly orally for 5 days, tablets Metronidazole 400 mg thrice daily orally for 5 days, tablets Fesolate 200 mg thrice daily orally for 6 weeks, tablets Folic acid 5 mg once daily for 6 weeks and tablets Vitamin C 200 mg thrice daily for 6 weeks. Her vital signs were monitored quarter-hourly for 2 hours, half-hourly for 4 hours, and thereafter 6 hourly. They remained normal. Oxytocin was discontinued after 4 hours, and the patient did not bleed from the vagina. She was fed immediately after recovery from anaesthesia.

24 hours on admission:

The patient had recovered from anaesthesia and had no complaints. She was afebrile and was not pale. Her pulse rate was 80 beats per minute with a regular rhythm and full volume; her blood pressure was 110/80 mmHg, and her heart sounds were normal. The uterus was well contracted and was compatible with 16 weeks gestation. She was draining normal lochia. She had also commenced breastfeeding, and the baby was suckling satisfactorily.

2nd - 4th day of admission:

The patient continued making significant progress and was discharged on the fourth day of admission. Her packed cell volume was 30%. She was in a stable condition and eating adequately; therefore, she was given a 6-week appointment at the post-natal clinic.

Immediately after discharge, her baby received BCG and Hepatitis vaccination at the pediatric clinic. The baby was also scheduled for subsequent immunizations in 6 weeks.

Follow-up:

She was seen at the post-natal clinic with her baby and husband for her six-week appointment. She and her baby were in good health; she was exclusively breastfeeding her baby and was lactating adequately. The baby weighed 5.5 kg. The baby had received the scheduled immunization for 6 weeks and booked for subsequent ones.

Lochia had ceased, and she was yet to commence her menstrual flow. Her PCV was 33%, and her urinalysis showed normal parameters. Abdominal examination showed a uterine size of about 12 weeks. The patient was counseled on the risks involved in childbirth in a facility lacking relevant skilled birth attendants. She was also educated on contraception and the recurrent nature of retained placenta and advised to seek tertiary supervision in subsequent deliveries.

Summary:

A 31-year-old woman was diagnosed with retained placenta following delivery at a maternity home despite having received antenatal care at the hospital. Manual removal of the placenta under anaesthesia was done.

Discussion:

Retained placenta refers to a failure to completely deliver the placenta within 30 minutes to one hour after the delivery of the baby.[1-3] Immediately following the delivery of a baby, contractions occur which result in spontaneous detachment of the placenta from the uterine wall and its subsequent delivery. Failure of this to occur results in retained placenta. This patient presented with a failure to deliver the placenta about an hour after the delivery of her baby. Retained placenta is a common cause of post-partum hemorrhage, both primary and secondary.[2,3] It is a potentially life-threatening condition and affects 0.5-3.3% of women following normal deliveries.[3] Risk factors include multiparity, uterine atony, fibroids, previous placental retention, home delivery, and mismanaged third stage of labour.[3,4] The likely risk factor in the index patient was mismanaged third stage of labor, which occurred because she had delivered in a maternity home with poor medical facilities and personnel. The gold standard of management includes adequate emergency resuscitation and manual removal of the placenta under anesthesia.[3] Other methods include the use of uterotonic drugs with controlled cord traction, umbilical vein injection of saline solution, and nitroglycerin.[3,5] Manual removal of the placenta was done for the index patient with a resultant good outcome.

It was noteworthy that though this patient had booked for antenatal care in a proper health facility and kept all her antenatal clinic appointments, she went on to be delivered in a maternity home. Maternal health-seeking behavior is a major influence on pregnancy outcomes,[6] as good health-seeking behavior by pregnant women has been associated with positive pregnancy outcomes.[6] Health-seeking behavior has been defined as any action or inaction undertaken by individuals who perceive themselves to have a health problem or to be ill for the purpose of finding an appropriate remedy.[7] Thus, maternal health-seeking behavior during pregnancy has been regarded as the way mothers take care of their health and that of the unborn child in order for both to remain healthy throughout pregnancy.[6]

Different factors influence the health-seeking behaviors of pregnant women. They could be socio-demographic factors like maternal age, parity, occupation, education, and distance to health facility;[8] socio-economic factors like cost of care, income, type, and severity of illness could also influence maternal health-seeking behaviours,[7,8] and cultural factors such as male dominance in decision-making; cultural norms, and religious beliefs.[7,8] The influence of religion has fueled the patronage of faith-based providers as there are strong beliefs that supernatural factors have the potential to influence pregnancy outcomes.[9,10] This was the situation with the index patient who resorted to a faith-based maternity home for delivery.

Lessons learned/Recommendations:

Family physicians should advocate for targeted health messages aimed at reducing knowledge gaps. They should also promote health education and empower pregnant women during antenatal clinics. This approach will help dispel harmful cultural myths surrounding childbirth.

References

1. Yusuf SC, Panti AA, Nnadi DC. An appraisal of retained placenta in Sokoto: a five-year review. Orient Journal of Medicine. 2013; 25: 1-2

2. Cheung WM., Hawkes A, Ibish, S, Weeks, AD. The retained placenta: historical and geographical rate variations. Journal of Obstetrics and Gynecology. 2011; 31:37.

3. Iklaki, C, Emechebe C, Njoku C, Ago B and Ugwu B. Socio-demographic profile and complications of patients with the retained placenta in a tertiary center, South-South Nigeria. *Open Access Library Journal*, **3**, 1-8.

4. Zmora I. Risk factors, early and late postpartum complications of retained placenta: A case control study. European Journal of Obstetrics and Gynecology and Reproductive Biology. 2019; 236: 160 – 165

5. Abdel-Aleem H, Abdel-Aleem MA, Shaaban OM. Nitroglycerin for management of retained placenta. Cochrane Database of Systematic Reviews. 2015;11

6. Ehiemere IO. Maternal health seeking behavior and pregnancy outcomes in rural communities in Enugu State, Southeast Nigeria. Journal of Community Medicine and Health Education. 2016; 6:3

7. Latunji OO, Akinyemi OO. Factors influencing health-seeking behavior among civil servants in Ibadan, Nigeria. Ann Ib Postgrad Med. 2018; 16(1):52–60.

8. Egbuniwe MC, Egboka OL, Nwankwo UC. Health-seeking behavior amongst pregnant women attending antenatal clinic in primary health care centers in rural communities of Nnewi North L.G.A Anambra State. J. Res Nurs Midwifery 2016;5(1):1-10

9. Akeju DO, Oladapo OT, Vidler M, Akinmade AA, Sawchuck D, Qureshi R et al. Determinants of health

care seeking behavior during pregnancy in Ogun State, Nigeria. Reproductive Health. 2016;13(1):32

10. Al-Mujtaba M, Cornelius LJ, Galadanci H, Erekaha S, Okundaye JN, Adeyemi OA et al. Evaluating religious influences on the utilization of maternal health services among Muslim and Christian women in North-Central Nigeria. Biomed Res Int. 2016; 2016:3645415. doi 10.1155/2016/3645415.

Chapter Seven

Foreign Body In The Ear

A 25-year-old female trader was seen at the Outpatient Clinic with complaints of discomfort in the right ear of eight hours' duration. The patient was apparently well until eight hours prior to presentation when a sensation of movement within her right ear woke her up from sleep. Her right ear felt heavy, as though an object was lodged inside it. She had not had this sensation before retiring to bed the night before. She initially tilted her ear to the side, trying to see if the object would fall out, but there was no relief. Following this, she used a broomstick to try to clean her right ear, and when this was unsuccessful, she put some drops of palm kernel oil into her ear. The movement sensation became worse, and she had such extreme discomfort in the ear that she could no longer sleep for the rest of the night. There was no ear pain, no ear discharge, and no abnormal sounds in her right ear. Also, she did not have any symptoms in the left ear. These symptoms made the patient visit the hospital as soon as it was daybreak; she was worried that she would become deaf in that ear even more so as she had received a prophecy in church some weeks earlier that a negative event would occur in her life. She wanted a proper examination of her ear and the removal of any object within her ear.

She had previously been treated for Pulmonary Tuberculosis at the Infectious Disease Hospital five years prior to this visit and had completed her drug regimen. She had no history of hypertension, diabetes, asthma, or sickle cell disease.

She was the fourth child in a polygamous home where her father had three wives, two unmarried girlfriends who had children for him, and about 17 children. Her parents lived in the village while she resided alone in a single room in the city. She had dropped out of secondary school due to financial hardship and was a petty trader dealing in farm products. She shared toilet facilities (water cistern) with two other tenants and drank borehole water. She was intimately involved with a taxi driver and regularly indulged in both protected and unprotected sexual intercourse. She also consumed alcoholic beverages (beer, spirits, and palm wine) occasionally. She did not take tobacco in any form.

A general physical examination showed an anxious-looking woman who was not febrile, pale, cyanosed, or icteric. There was no peripheral lymphadenopathy or pedal oedema. Examination of her left ear did not reveal any abnormalities, but examination of the right ear showed mild tenderness of the pinna and a blackish oily substance on the pinna. Gentle cleaning of the external auditory canal with cotton wool and probe yielded the same blackish oily substance and cerumen. Otoscopic examination revealed the carcass of a cockroach within the auditory canal, partially obscuring the tympanic membrane. In the Rinne test, air conduction was better than bone conduction in both ears as she heard the vibrating tuning fork sound when it was placed in front of her pinna. This signified a positive (or normal) Rinne test. In the Weber test, the patient heard the vibrating tuning fork sound equally in both ears signifying a normal Weber test. There were no abnormalities of the nose and throat upon examination.

Her pulse rate was 74 beats per minute, full volume, with a regular rhythm that synchronized with other peripheral pulses. Her blood pressure was 130/70 mmHg; the first and second heart sounds only were heard. Her respiratory rate was 18 cycles per minute; she had vesicular breath sounds, and her chest was clinically clear. Examination of other systems did not reveal any abnormalities.

A diagnosis of an organic foreign body in the right ear canal was made.

Management:

The diagnosis, examination findings, and management principles were fully explained to the patient. She was told that an insect was within her ear, and this was the reason for the discomfort she felt. Thus, it had to be removed. The patient was told that it would be removed by manual extraction. She was concerned that the procedure would involve surgery, and she did not want to be anesthetized or undergo surgery. She was, however, reassured that the procedure would be done right there in the clinic without anesthesia. She consented, and manual extraction of the insect was carried out.

The procedure involved the use of the following equipment: disposable gloves, cotton tips, receptacle (kidney dish), alligator forceps, and headlamp. Before the procedure, it was ascertained by the patient that there was no longer any movement within her ear. This was because the insect had been killed when the patient introduced a mineral oil (palm kernel oil) into her ear. She was seated comfortably, and both ears were re-examined with an otoscope. Having confirmed the location and depth of the foreign body, the tip of the pinna was grasped and pulled upwards. A pair of alligator forceps was then introduced into the ear and advanced through the external auditory canal until it reached the edge of the insect. This edge was then grasped with the forceps, and the entire insect was pulled out of the ear canal. Examination of the insect revealed a cockroach. Subsequently, the right ear was examined again to ensure that all insect debris had been removed as well as to examine the now-visible tympanic membrane. The tympanic membrane was intact and there were no abnormalities or abrasions within the ear canal. Ear toileting was then done using cotton tips. Following the procedure, tablets of Diclofenac potassium 50mg, as needed for 2 days orally, were prescribed for the patient, and she was asked to return to the clinic in one week. She was advised not to insert any foreign objects into her ears or to instil any ear drops into her ears.

Follow-up:

When seen a week later, she had no complaints. However, she was worried about how an insect had found its way into her ear. Thus, she was educated on the importance of good hygiene in the home as a major pillar of infection prevention and good health. The patient was educated in home hygiene practices which included food hygiene, personal hygiene, proper waste disposal and adequate sanitation, and pest control. She was told that poor hygiene within the home could lead to many preventable infectious diseases as well as the kind of medical condition that made her present to the hospital. Considering that the patient had previously suffered from Tuberculosis, which is an infection linked to overcrowded, unsanitary conditions, a home visit was scheduled two days after the clinic visit to assess the sanitary state of the patient's home and properly counsel her.

Home visit:

The home visit revealed the extremely poor sanitary state of the patient's home. She lived in a single room which was overcrowded with home furniture, old appliances and the farm products she traded in. The room showed evidence of not having been cleaned in a long while. To this, the patient responded that she was too busy attending to her business. The patient was counselled to decongest her living space by clearing out old useless items and constructing a wooden cupboard for her farm produce, which she would keep outside her door. Decongesting her living space would ensure that no insects or rodents would occupy it. An inspection of the toilet facility, which she shared with two co-tenants, also revealed poor sanitary conditions; she was advised to team up with her co-tenants to adequately clean and disinfect the toilet facility in order to prevent toilet infections, diarrheal diseases, and vector-borne diseases.

A second home visit was made a week later, and it was apparent that the patient had adhered to all the counsel which she had been given. Her home was well cleaned and now more spacious due to being decongested; her toilet had been washed and disinfected with Izal disinfectant. She was commended for her efforts and advised to maintain hygienic practices.

Summary:

A 25-year-old female trader was diagnosed with a foreign body in the right ear, which turned out to be a cockroach. The cockroach was manually removed, and she was counseled on the importance of good hygiene. This health education was reinforced by home visits.

Discussion:

A foreign body in the ear could be described as any object within the ear, other than cerumen that can cause harm by its mere presence if immediate medical attention is not sought.[1,2] It is a common otorhinolaryngology emergency seen in outpatient clinics and the Emergency Room accounting for as high as 11% of cases seen in ENT services.[3] The index patient presented with a foreign body within her right ear.

The entry of a foreign body into the ear can be intentional or unintentional. Intentional cases usually occur when people use objects with detachable parts, such as cotton buds or match sticks, to clean or scratch their ears.[4] Unintentional entry could occur from accidental causes like road traffic injuries and missile injuries; mental illnesses like schizophrenia, bipolar disorder, and mental retardation,[5,6] and also in cases where live insects crawl into the ear.[4] The patient presented to the clinic because an insect had crawled into her ear while she was sleeping at night, thus making her case an unintentional entry of a foreign body.

Ear foreign bodies are of different forms and, as such, have been classified within various categories. These categories include organic or inorganic, animate or inanimate, metallic or non-metallic, hygroscopic or non-hygroscopic.[4,7] Authors have reported the removal of objects like beads, cotton tips, seeds, garlic, papers, button batteries, blue tooth devices, and insects from patients' ears.[4,5] In the case of the index patient, a cockroach, which is an organic foreign body, was extracted from her ear.

The type of foreign body extracted can give a strong pointer to the immediate environment of the patient.[8] In children, it is not uncommon to find beads, tiny toy parts, erasers, and other items found in the school environment within the ear canal. Likewise, in this patient's case, the presence of an insect within the ear reflected the unhygienic state of her environment as such health education on environmental sanitation was offered to this patient, with the physician going further to conduct a home visit to properly guide her and prevent recurrence of her health condition.

The clinical management of this condition necessitates the removal of the foreign object, and the method of removal often depends on the type of foreign body involved. Techniques for removal include manual instrumentation, irrigation, suction, and cyanoacrylate.[1,6] Removal of live insects involves killing and immobilizing the insect with mineral oil before removal by manual extraction.[6] Beads are not easily graspable and thus removed by using a right-angle hook, which is used for spherical objects or by using cyanoacrylate (superglue) on the wooden end of a cotton-tipped applicator.

Manual extraction of the insect was the procedure adopted in the case of the index patient. However, it has been found that many people engage in home management of ear foreign bodies before even presenting at the hospital.[7,9] The use of mineral oil is also a home management technique for the removal of foreign insect bodies and was even applied by the patient when she put palm kernel oil into her ear to sense movement within the ear.

Other home management procedures include the use of sharp objects to remove the foreign body and vigorous shaking of the ear.[7,9] These procedures can lead to complications like tympanic membrane perforation, lacerations, and hearing impairments.[10]

Finally, to ensure holistic and comprehensive management of this patient since she had volunteered a social history which showed that she regularly engaged in unprotected sexual intercourse, she was counselled on the importance of safer sex practices, which were abstinence, avoidance of multiple sexual partners and the use of condoms during sexual intercourse. There is a need for family physicians to use every available opportunity for sex education to prevent sexually transmitted infections, which increases the disease and economic burden on the patient and family.

Lessons learned/Recommendations:

Family physicians should be well trained in the relevant skills needed to remove ear foreign bodies. Patients should be educated on preventive ways of avoiding this problem and the need to desist from removal of foreign bodies using unorthodox measures.

References

1. Parajuli R. Foreign bodies in the ear, nose, and throat: an experience in a tertiary care hospital in central Nepal. *Int Arch Otorhinolaryngol.* 2014; 19(2):121-123.

2. Sarkar S, Roychoudhury A, Roychaudhuri B K. Foreign bodies in ENT in a teaching hospital in Eastern India. Indian J Otolaryngol Head Neck Surg. 2010; 62(2):118-120.

3. Silva BSR, Souza LO, Camera MG, Tamiso AGB, Castanheira LVR. Foreign bodies in otorhinolaryngology: a study of 128 cases. Int Arch Otorhinolaryngol. 2009;13(4):394-9.

4. Al-Juboori AN. Aural foreign bodies: Descriptive study of 224 patients in al-fallujah general hospital, Iraq. *Int J Otolaryngol.* 2013; 2013:401289.

5. Shrestha I, Shrestha B L, Amatya R CM. Analysis of ear, nose, and throat foreign bodies in Dhulikhel

hospital. Kathmandu Univ Med J (KUMJ) 2012; 10(38):4–8.

6. Olajuyin O, Olatunya OS. Aural foreign body extraction in children: a double-edged sword. *Pan Afr Med J.* 2015; 20:186.

7. Adedeji TO, Sogebi OA, Bande S. Clinical spectrum of ear, nose, and throat foreign bodies in Northwestern Nigeria. *Afr Health Sci.* 2016; 16(1):292–297.

8. United Nations. Water, sanitation, and hygiene. 2015. Available at https://www.unwater.org/water-facts/water-sanitation-and-hygiene/

9. Amutta SB, Iseh KR, Aliyu D, Abdullahi M, Abdulrahman GA. Ear, nose, and throat foreign bodies in a tertiary institution in Sokoto, Nigeria. Sahel Med J. 2013; 16:87-92

10. Olajide TG, Ologe FE, Arigbede OO. Management of foreign bodies in the ear: A retrospective review of 123

cases in Nigeria. *Ear Nose Throat J.* 2011; 90(11): E169.

Chapter Eight

Chronic Leg Ulcer Due To Varicose Veins

A 51-year-old traffic warden was seen at the clinic with a wound on the left leg of 8 months duration, pain and swelling of the left leg of 2 weeks duration. She was apparently well until 8 months before the presentation when she noticed swellings on her left leg. These swellings were small, painful, itchy, and occurred as lines along her left leg. There was a blackish discoloration on the leg.

The swellings eventually ruptured to leave wounds that drained pus and fluid. There was pain in the lower part of the same leg. The pain was sharp, continuous, radiated to her left thigh, and was severe enough to restrict her mobility. She felt relief from the pain after she had taken pain relievers for some days. There was, however progressive enlargement of her left leg and the wound. She has had a positive history of standing for long hours on her job (about 8 – 10 hours) for the past twelve years. For her symptoms, she had sought treatment at a patent drug store, consulted a traditional healer for herbal remedies, and visited a nurse occasionally who dressed the wound.

Two weeks before the presentation, she suffered a fall, which resulted in a wound breakdown, as well as severe continuous pain in her left leg. This necessitated her visit to the hospital. She feared that her leg would be amputated since the wound was extensive. She strongly believed that she had unknowingly stepped on evil charms placed on a public road, which caused her symptoms. Her functionality was impaired as she found it difficult to walk without assistance. She expected to be cured of her illness and, more importantly, have cosmesis restored to her left leg.

In her past medical and surgical history, there was no history of hypertension, diabetes, epilepsy, sickle cell disease, or asthma. There was also no history of previous surgeries or blood transfusions.

She was Para $2^{+\ 0}$ and had been menopausal for two years. Her children were delivered through vaginal delivery. She had never done a Pap smear.

The patient was the third of seven children (3 males and 4 females). Her mother was alive, but her father was deceased, having died at old age. She volunteered that having prominent veins on the leg was part of her family ancestry, as her father and sisters had similar conditions. She worked with the Nigerian Police Force as a traffic warden. The patient was separated from her husband. Her children, one female aged 22 years and one male aged 19 years, were students at a tertiary institution (University of Calabar). She took alcohol occasionally and did not take tobacco in any form. Her family APGAR assessment was

7/10, indicating a moderately dysfunctional family. The family was at Stage 6 (launching center family) of Evelyn Duvall's staging. The source of healthcare finance was the National Health Insurance Scheme (NHIS).

She had no urinary symptoms, increased thirst, weight loss, hot flushes, abnormal vaginal bleeding or masses, headache, cough, or difficulty in breathing.

She was assisted into the consulting room by her son and was in pain. She weighed 90kg with a height of 1.65 meters and a BMI of $33.05 kg/m^2$, signifying Class 1 obesity. Her femoral lymph nodes were enlarged. There was oedema of the left leg.

Peripheral venous examination:

The right leg had no abnormalities. Her left leg was markedly enlarged with hyperpigmentation of the skin. There was varicosity of the veins on the upper two-thirds of the left leg. An ulcer measuring 8 cm in width and 6 cm in length was present at the lateral malleolus of the left leg. It had sloping edges, and the floor was covered by pus and necrotic debris. The surrounding skin was tender and warmer than other areas of the lower limb. There was no loss of sensation on any part of the left leg, and peripheral pulses were present. There was restriction of movement at the left ankle joint due to pain, and passive inversion, plantar flexion, and extension elicited tenderness.

The Trendelenburg test revealed there was tortuosity of veins above the ulcer when the left leg was brought down, which was evidence of varicosity.

Her pulse rate was 72 beats per minute with a regular rhythm and normal volume. There was synchrony of all peripheral pulses. The dorsal pedis pulses in both feet were present and had a regular rhythm and normal volume. Her blood pressure was 120/70 mmHg; the apex beat was at the fifth left intercostal space on the mid-clavicular line. There was no distension of her neck veins, and the jugular venous pressure was not raised. The first and second heart sounds were heard on auscultation. Her respiratory rate was 18 cycles per minute, chest expansion was equal, percussion notes were resonant, and breath sounds were vesicular. Examination of other systems revealed normal findings.

A provisional diagnosis of Chronic leg ulcer due to venous insufficiency in a patient with Grade 1 obesity to exclude diabetic foot ulcer, chronic osteomyelitis, and malignancy was made.

Management:

The diagnosis and management plan that was to be adopted in her treatment was discussed with the patient. The management plan involved surgical debridement and review by the Plastic surgeon for skin graft and wound dressing. Her fears were allayed when she was told that her left leg would not be amputated, but in due course, healing would occur, and her leg would be restored to normal aesthesis. Emphasis was put on adherence to treatment as a means of achieving optimal healing outcomes. She was informed that her illness was not due to evil charms but was likely due to a combination of obesity, her job, which entailed standing for long hours, and a family history of varicose veins. She was admitted and booked for surgical debridement and biopsy of the ulcer the following day.

Laboratory investigations included complete blood count (CBC), urine analysis, fasting blood glucose (FBG), human immunodeficiency virus (HIV) screening, wound swab for microscopy, culture, and sensitivity (M/C/S) and plain radiograph of the distal one-third of the left leg in the anteroposterior and lateral positions. A Doppler ultrasound scan was requested; however, it was declined by the patient due to the high cost and her financial limitations, as the test was not covered by the National Health Insurance Scheme. The results obtained showed urinalysis results had normal values, packed cell volume was 32%, Hb 10.6g/dl, WBC

9.5 x 10^3 with differentials of neutrophils 39%, lymphocytes 51% and eosinophil 10%.

The Erythrocyte sedimentation rate was 16 mm/hour, and fasting blood glucose was 4.8mmol/l. Wound swab microscopy, culture, and sensitivity yielded growth of *Staphylococcus aureus* sensitive to cloxacillin, ampicillin-cloxacillin, ciprofloxacin, and levofloxacin. HIV screening was non-reactive. The radiograph result showed an intact left tibia/fibula. There were no lytic lesions, periosteal thickening, loss of trabecular architecture, or sequestrum formation. This excluded the absence of chronic osteomyelitis.

A definitive diagnosis of chronic leg ulcer due to varicose veins was made.

She was given intravenous ceftriaxone 1 gram daily for 1-week, intravenous metronidazole 500 milligrams 8 hourly for 1-week, intravenous gentamicin 80 mg 8 hourly for 1 week, tablets ibuprofen 400 milligrams 12 hourly for 5 days, and tablets vitamin C 200 milligrams three times daily for 2 weeks. The ulcer was cleaned and dressed, and the left leg was elevated. The procedure of surgical debridement was explained to her, and informed consent was obtained.

Debridement:

Surgical debridement of the ulcer was done in the theatre under general anaesthesia. With the patient supine, the skin was cleaned and draped. The surface of the ulcer was irrigated with a normal saline solution and then probed with forceps to determine the depth and locate any foreign matter. Biopsy samples were obtained from the margin and floor of the ulcer and sent for histopathological analysis. Necrotic tissue was cut off until healthy bleeding tissue was reached, and subsequently, the ulcer was irrigated using a normal saline solution. The wound was dressed in layers using tulle gras (sofratulle) dressing, povidone iodine, and gauze. A crepe bandage was applied firmly over the dressing. She was to be nursed in the ward with her left leg elevated and the ulcer dressed daily. She was excused from duty for one week in the first instance.

1st week post admission:

In the days following the debridement, the patient initially complained of pain and pruritus in her left leg, which gradually reduced with each passing day. The wound was dressed daily. After one week, the wound surface was clean with minimal healthy granulation tissue seen on some areas of the ulcer surface. She remained on admission for another week, being nursed with her leg elevated. She was placed on tablets of acetaminophen 1000mg, tablets of ampicillin-cloxacillin 500mg six hourly, and tablets of levofloxacin 750mg daily for a week. Histopathological analysis results showed no evidence of malignancy.

Two weeks post-admission:

After two weeks, the wound site was clean with healthy granulation tissue covering the surface of the wound, the edges of the wound were smooth, and the wound diameter had reduced. She was discharged and scheduled for alternate day wound dressings. She was asked to reduce her activities to the minimum required and keep her leg elevated when sitting or lying down.

A compression bandage was prescribed for her to be worn during the day and removed at night. This was to aid the healing of the varicose veins. Crutches were prescribed to prevent her from bearing weight on her left leg. She was also counseled on appropriate dietary measures to aid weight reduction, and a dietary plan was formulated. These included a reduction of carbohydrates, fats, and oils as well as an increased intake of fiber-rich foods, poultry, and fish. Oral Vitamin C tablets 200mg three times daily were continued for one week. She was issued a medical report for her employers and a one-week sick leave, which was renewed on a weekly basis for four weeks.

The patient was referred to the plastic surgeon for co-management of the chronic leg ulcer. The plastic surgeon reviewed her and recommended her for skin graft surgery. Prior to the surgery, 3% sodium tetradecyl sulphate, a sclerosant, was injected into the varicose veins to treat the varicosity and prevent recurrence.

Skin graft surgery:

A skin graft was obtained from the ipsilateral limb where the ulcer was located at the lateral aspect of the thigh under aseptic conditions. There were no complications during surgery. The recipient site was inspected on the sixth day post-surgery. It was dry and had no swelling or redness. Subsequently, wet dressing using saline-soaked gauze was done on alternate days until the graft site healed. The donor site was opened on the 21st day post-surgery. It had healed considerably. It was left open with daily applications of Vaseline cream on the surface.

Follow-up:

At her first follow-up visit a month later, she had no new complaints. The skin graft site was healing without complications. She was mobilizing well with her crutches. She had adhered to the dietary plan and now weighed 83kg. A sick leave of four weeks had been granted by her employers and her general condition was satisfactory. Following a collaboration between the author and the medical superintendent of the police clinic, her role as a traffic warden was changed to a desk officer to aid her recovery.

Within three months, there was marked healing of the skin graft site. There was a marked shrinking of the varicose veins. She was to continue using the compression bandage but discontinued from wound dressing and crutches.

Subsequently, she was discharged from the outpatient clinic.

Summary:

A 51-year-old female traffic warden was diagnosed with chronic leg ulcer due to varicose veins. She had the belief that her illness was because she had stepped on charms. These beliefs were addressed through health education, and she was managed with surgical debridement, skin graft, and medications. Dietary counseling was also done.

Discussion:

A chronic leg ulcer is defined as a defect in the skin below the level of the knee, persisting for more than six weeks and showing no tendency to heal after three or more months.[1] The index patient had a leg ulcer that had persisted for about eight months and showed no tendency to heal, thereby fulfilling the criteria for diagnosis as a chronic leg ulcer.

Chronic leg ulcers are an important clinical condition affecting approximately 1% of the adult population and 0.6 - 3% of people older than 65 years of age, increasing to about 5% in people aged over 80 years.[1,2] A study by the Wound Healing Society in the United States showed that about 15% of older adults in the United States suffer from chronic leg ulcers, predominantly varicose leg ulcers, pressure ulcers (bed sores), and diabetic leg ulcers.[1,3]

The common causes include trauma, venous disease, arterial disease, and neuropathy,[3] with less common causes being metabolic disorders, haematological disorders, and infective disorders.[3,4] Varicose veins are twisted, dilated veins most commonly located on the lower extremities.[5] Risk factors for the development of varicosity include chronic cough, constipation, and family history of venous disease, female sex, obesity, older age, pregnancy, and prolonged standing.[5] The index patient was an overweight female traffic warden whose job necessitated prolonged standing over long periods and a family history of varicose veins. Diabetes mellitus as a cause was excluded because she had normal blood glucose results, and the absence of bony involvement or sinuses excluded chronic osteomyelitis. Arterial cause was also excluded because they are usually associated with cardiac or cerebrovascular disease as well as abnormal pedal pulses.

In spite of the etiology being understood, cultural perceptions still abound with widespread beliefs that these ulcers are caused by people stepping on evil charms placed on public roads and also that effective treatment necessitates traditional methods or herbal remedies.[6,7]

The patient believed that her illness was due to evil charms placed on a public road, which she had stepped on, and had tried herbal interventions before seeking medical care. Thus, she was properly educated on the likely cause and risk factors of her illness and disabused of the wrong perceptions that she had.

Diagnosis of chronic leg ulcers usually depends on identifying the underlying pathophysiology, but the clinical course of the ulcer can suggest its aetiology.[7,8] As such, in this patient various investigations were done to identify the etiology of her ulcer.

The Doppler ultrasonography, which is important in the diagnosis of venous ulcers, was not done, however, due to the patient's financial constraints.

Treatment of chronic leg ulcers can be achieved through medical and surgical measures.[8,9,10] These include surgical debridement, compression therapy, lifestyle changes, and preventative care such as health education.[8,9,10] All these were utilized in the treatment of the index patient to provide patient-centered care. She was also properly educated regarding the aesthesis of her leg to improve her self-image.

Lessons Learned/Recommendations:

In this part of the world, there are strong beliefs on the spiritual causes of chronic ulcers. Health education on the etiology of chronic ulcers by family physicians is important because of the strong belief in the supernatural causes of these ulcers.

References

1. Shubhangi VA. Chronic leg ulcers: epidemiology, etiopathogenesis, and management. Ulcers 2013; 17:4:1

2. Eftychia P, Anargyros K, Christos C. Psychosocial aspects in patients with chronic leg ulcers. Wounds 2017; 29(10):306–310.

3. Lauren C, Samina S. Diagnosis, and treatment of venous ulcer. Am Fam Physician. 2010; 81(8):989-996.

4. Ruettermann M, Maier-Hasselmann A, Nink-Grebe B, Burckhardt M. Local treatment of chronic wounds in patients with peripheral vascular disease, chronic venous insufficiency, and diabetes. Deutsches Ärzteblatt international. 2013;110: 25-31

5. Newton H. Leg ulcers: differences between venous and arterial. Wounds Essentials. 2011; 6(1): 1:20–28

6. Siddiqui AR, Bernstein JM. Chronic wound infection: facts and controversies. Clinics in Dermatology. 2010;28(5):519–526

7. Nwafor FI, Tchimene MK, Onyekere PK, Nweze NO. Ethnobiological study of traditional medicine practices for the treatment of chronic leg ulcer in South-Eastern Nigeria. Journal of plants science. 2018;3(1)

8. Kahle B, Hermanns AJ, Gallenkemper G. Evidence-based treatment of chronic leg ulcers. Deutsches Ärzteblatt International. 2011; 108(14):231–237

9. Sasanka CS. Venous ulcers of the lower limb: where do we stand? Indian Journal of Plastic Surgery. 2012; 45(2):266–274

10. Rahman GA, Adigun IA, Fadeyi A. Epidemiology, aetiology, and treatment of chronic leg ulcer: experience with sixty patients. Annals of African Medicine. 2010;9(1):1–4

Chapter Nine

Left Dorsal Wrist Ganglion In A 28-Year-Old Woman

A 28-year-old female engineer presented at the General Hospital with complaints of a lump on the left wrist of 8 months duration.

The patient was apparently well until 8 months before she presented at the hospital when she noticed a lump on her left wrist. It was gradual in onset and progressively increased in size slowly. The lump was painless and initially did not affect the function of her left forearm, but a few weeks before her visit, she started feeling discomfort anytime she worked on the computer. There was no history of trauma or insect bites prior to the onset of her symptoms; however, she noticed that the lump first appeared at the time she was nursing her baby. There was no history of similar swellings on other parts of her body, weight loss, or numbness of the extremities.

At the onset of her symptoms, she frequently massaged the lump using hot water and balms. She also took antibiotics for a long time because she assumed it was a 'boil,' but the lump did not disappear. She further sought the advice of a friend who was a doctor and was told that the lump would require surgical removal or it may disappear as time progressed. She decided not to have surgery because she had recently had an emergency Caesarean operation with complications and so was averse to surgery. However, the lump did not regress but rather increased in size until it distorted the appearance of her wrist and affected her work. Having read on the internet that a lump could undergo a cancerous transformation, she became afraid, and this prompted her to present to the clinic. Her expectation was that the lump would be surgically removed but without general or spinal anesthesia. The lump affected her function as it caused her much discomfort, thus limiting her work. There was no cough, difficulty in breathing, excessive urination, increased thirst, or increased consumption of water.

In her past medical and surgical history, she had no history of hypertension, epilepsy, asthma, diabetes, or sickle cell disease. She had undergone an emergency Caesarean operation for obstructed labor over a year before her clinic visit. She experienced complications like surgical wound breakdown and spinal headache, which lasted for about three weeks after surgery. There was no history of drug allergy, and she was not on any routine medications.

She was about 11 years old when menarche began. Her menstrual periods lasted 4 days, and her menstrual cycle was 28-30 days. She was $P1^{+0}$, and she had a 15-month-old daughter who had been delivered through a Caesarean operation. There was a history of dysmenorrhea. She used Billing's method as a contraceptive measure.

She was the second child in a family of five children, 2 females and 3 males. Her parents and siblings were all alive and well. Her mother was a known hypertensive patient. There was no family history of similar lumps. She was married to a 35-year-old marketing officer working at a commercial bank and they had one female child. They lived in a rented two-bedroom apartment. She was a software engineer and owned a business center/cybercafé, which had three staff. The family APGAR score was 10/10, indicating a highly functional family and their source of healthcare financing was out-of-pocket.

The physical examination showed a young woman who was conscious, alert and well-oriented in time, person and place. She was afebrile (temperature 37.2^{0}C), not pale, anicteric, not cyanotic, and had no peripheral lymphadenopathy or pedal oedema. She had a feminine appearance with normal muscle bulk. Her right hand was normal, but she had a mass on the dorsal part of her left wrist near the scapholunate joint. It was oval and measured about 4x3 centimeters (cm). The mass was cystic, non-tender, mobile, and with no differential warmth. It trans-illuminated with a pen light. Motor and sensory examination was normal in all limbs.

There was no sign of meningeal irritation or cranial nerve deficit. Motor and sensory systems were normal. Her pulse rate was 80 beats per minute with a full volume and regular rhythm. The blood pressure was 120/70 mmHg, jugular venous pressure was not raised, and the apex beat was at the fifth left intercostal space on the mid-clavicular line. The first and second heart sounds were heard. The rate was 16 cycles per minute. Chest expansion was normal on both sides. There was good air entry with vesicular breath sounds. Examination of other systems did not reveal any abnormalities.

A diagnosis of the left dorsal wrist ganglion was made. The differential diagnoses included lipoma, tenosynovitis, epidermoid inclusion cyst, and intraneural cyst.

Management:

The diagnosis and management plan were fully explained to the patient. She was told that the lump would be excised from her wrist, and in agreement with her, she was booked for surgery a week after her clinic visit. This was to give her adequate time to prepare herself physically and mentally as well as to organize her family, home, and office in preparation for the days she would not be functioning. The investigations requested were packed cell volume (PCV), urine analysis, and HIV screening. The results showed PCV of 36% and normal parameters of urine analysis. HIV screening was non-reactive. On the proposed day of surgery, she presented at the clinic with her husband. An informed consent was obtained from her. She had no new complaints, and the examination did not reveal any abnormalities of her systems.

Procedure:

In the theatre, the patient was placed supine with the left upper limb abducted and placed on an arm board. A tourniquet was applied to the lower third of her left arm. Anesthesia was achieved using the Bier block. The skin of the dorsum of her left wrist extending to the mid-forearm was cleaned with 0.2% Chlorhexidine solution and draped. The margin of the mass was then marked with a temporary marker ink. A transverse skin incision was made with a scalpel over the apex of the mass, extending beyond both ends by 1cm. Dissection was done through the superficial fascia and extensor retinaculum to access the mass. It was excised, the tourniquet was released, and the dead space was apposed using chromic catgut 2/0 suture. Skin closure was done with nylon 3/0 suture. The wound was cleaned with 10% Povidone iodine, and then sterile gauze and pressure strapping were applied. The cyst removed was shown to the patient and then sent for histological examination.

Following the procedure, she was admitted for 2 hours of observation. A review after two hours showed her in a stable clinical condition. She was advised to rest her hand and prevent the operation site from getting wet. Tablets Diclofenac 50mg eight hourly for three days was prescribed for her, and she was discharged. She was scheduled for a follow-up visit in three days.

First follow-up visit:

At her first follow-up visit, she complained of minimal pain at the operation site; however, she had normal clinical findings on examination. The wound dressing was clean and dry. Examination of the wound revealed that the wound was clean and dry with well-apposed edges. It was dressed in Povidone iodine ointment, and light gauze was applied on its surface.

She was also given a prescription for Acetaminophen tablets 1000 mg eight hourly orally for three days. Thereafter, she was scheduled for another follow-up after four days.

Second follow-up visit:

When seen on this visit, she had no new complaints. Examination of the wound showed a healed wound. The sutures were removed during this visit. She was advised to gently resume her activities while avoiding stress on the left hand. Subsequently, she was discharged.

Summary:

A 28-year-old female software engineer was diagnosed with a ganglion cyst on the left wrist. She had delayed treatment of the cyst until she read that there could be a malignant transformation leading to death, which prompted her to seek care. A surgical excision of the cyst was done for her with positive outcomes.

Discussion:

Ganglion cysts are fluid-filled swellings associated with a joint or tendon sheath[1,2] They can affect any joint of the hand, wrist, or foot, but the most common location is the dorsum of the wrist.[1,2] where they make up about 50-70% of tumors found in this area.[3,4] It is prevalent during the second and third decades of life and has also been found to have a higher prevalence among females than males.[1] The index patient was a 28-year old woman who developed a cystic lesion on the dorsum of her left wrist.

This tumor has been known to occur following varying degrees of trauma like contusions, twisting, and stretching injuries.[3] It has also been found commonly among gymnasts.[2,3] The clinical features include swelling, pain, paresthesia, and muscle weakness.[5] In many cases, however, the cyst could be asymptomatic. Some cysts may even remain hidden under the skin and are referred to as occult ganglion.[5] Physical examination typically reveals a soft mass with a cystic consistency to palpation that may transilluminate with a penlight.[6] The patient presented with paresthesia and a mass on the wrist that transilluminated with a penlight consequently leading to the diagnosis.

Diagnosis may be achieved through clinical examination, standard X-rays, ultrasound, and magnetic resonance imaging (MRI).[6,7] An X-ray may show features of degenerative joint disease, particularly in the proximal carpal row, however, it usually gives negative findings.[7] Ultrasound and magnetic resonance imaging are very useful in diagnosing occult lesions.[7] This patient's diagnosis was done through clinical examination.

Treatment can be conservative or through surgical means.[8,9] Conservative treatment of ganglion cysts in the hand and wrist can be initiated by the primary-care clinician. It includes reassurance, benign neglect, splinting, non-steroidal anti-inflammatory drugs (NSAIDs), and aspiration of the lesion.[9] A common misconception about ganglion cyst treatment is that hitting it with a heavy book like a Bible or object will shrink it, hence the reason it was referred to as 'Bible cyst' in the olden days.[10] Where conservative treatment fails, surgical intervention may be appropriate.[8,9] The patient decided to have a surgical excision because the mass disrupted her function as well as due to fear of malignant transformation. Patients' fears about ganglion cysts usually include bad cosmesis, loss of function, and malignant growth.[6] The patient, who was an IT consultant, had read articles on ganglion cysts and the possibility of malignant transformation and was deeply afraid. This offered an opportunity for extensive health education of the patient.

Lessons learned/Recommendations.

This case showed the importance of ensuring that patients are fully educated on their health conditions before informed consent is obtained and any procedure is carried out. This will help to forestall inappropriate convictions, which could negatively impact future care.

References

1. Suen M, Fung B, Lung CP. Treatment of ganglion cysts. ISRN Orthopedics. https://doi.org/10.1155/2013/940615.

2. Mofikoya BO, Anunobi CC, Ugburo AO. Hand tumours in Lagos, Nigeria: a clinicopathologic study. East and Central African Journal of Surgery. 2013; 18(3).

3. Ahn JH, Choy WS, Kim HY. Operative treatment for ganglion cysts of the foot and ankle. J Foot Ankle Surg 2010; 49(5): 442-5.

4. Rathod CM, Nemade AS, Badole CM. Treatment of dorsal wrist ganglia by transfixation technique. Niger J Clin Pract. 2011; 14:445-8

5. Sonnery-Cottet, B, Guimarães TM, Daggett M, Pic JB, Kajetanek C, de Padua VB, Thaunat M. Anterior cruciate ligament ganglion cyst treated under computed tomography–guided aspiration in a professional soccer

player. Orthopaedic Journal of Sports Medicine.2016; 4:5

6. Ashindoitiang JA. Preliminary report of the effectiveness of tetracycline sclerotherapy in the treatment of ganglion. Plastic Surgery International. 2012: Article ID 624209

7. Woitzik E, Kissel J. Ganglion cyst of the foot treated with electroacupuncture: A case report. *J Can Chiropr Assoc.* 2013;57(4):310–315.

8. Head L, Gencarrell JR, Allen M, Boyd KU. Wrist ganglion treatment: systematic review and meta-analysis. The Journal of Hand Surgery. 2015: 40(3): 546

9. Babayo UD, Bello US, Mohammed BS, Aliyu S. Silk suture technique: a simple, easy, effective treatment of wrist ganglion and review of literature. International Journal of Science and Research. 2014; 3:9

10. Trivedi NN, Schreiber JJ, Daluiski A. Blunt force may be an effective treatment for ganglion cysts. *HSS J.* 2016; 12 (2):100–104.

Chapter Ten

Severe Hypertension Due To Poor Adherence

A 44-year-old ward assistant presented to the outpatient clinic with a headache of a month duration and difficulty in sleeping for 2 weeks duration.

The patient was a known hypertensive who presented with a headache, which was generalized, dull, throbbing, intermittent, and usually occurring at any time of the day. It was relieved temporarily when she took analgesics like acetaminophen and aggravated by mobility. There was associated photophobia, dizziness, and nausea. There were no complaints of neck stiffness, vomiting or fever. She also complained of difficulty in initiating and maintaining sleep, which started about 2 weeks prior to presentation. She usually woke up in the morning feeling very exhausted. There was no history of cough, palpitations, difficulty in breathing, blurred vision, fainting attacks, or change in color and odor of urine. She did not have an increased frequency of micturition, increased thirst, or weight loss. There was no history of weakness in any part of the body, abdominal pain, pain on micturition, bleeding from the vagina, or vaginal discharge. She had no body swellings, breast masses or breast discharge, joint pain, or paresthesia.

She was diagnosed with hypertension about five years before presentation and had received medical care at the tertiary hospital where she worked for about two years but subsequently defaulted in follow-up. Her prescribed drug was Valsartan/hydrochlorothiazide (Co-Diovan) 80/12.5mg. However, she had stopped taking her antihypertensive medication due to a paucity of funds and had resorted to herbal remedies. She was afraid she would die from hypertension, just like her elder sister, who died from complications of a stroke. She had the idea that her symptoms were due to her incessant worrying over her husband's unemployment, which had left her as the sole breadwinner for their five children. The symptoms made her feel very ill and unable to work. She expected that her visit to the hospital would yield an improvement in her symptoms and physical state.

Her past medical and surgical history showed there was no history of asthma, epilepsy, diabetes, or sickle cell disease. There was also no history of previous surgeries or blood transfusions. In the obstetric and gynecological history, her last menstrual period occurred a week before she came to the hospital. She was not using any method of contraception.

Her family and social history showed that the patient was the third of five children, 2 females and 3 males. Both parents were alive. She had an elder sister who had died a year before the patient's visit from complications arising from hypertension. The patient was married to a 48-year-old former company worker who was now unemployed. She was a staff in a tertiary hospital. They had five children, 3 females and 2 males. Four of the children were school-age children, while the last child was a baby. Her source of health care financing was out of pocket. She was a non-smoker and took alcoholic drinks occasionally. The patient did not engage in a fitness routine and was not particular about her diet. On assessment of family function, the Apgar score was put at 6/10, indicative of a moderately dysfunctional family.

Her physical examination indicated she was anxious-looking, alert, not pale, anicteric, afebrile, not dehydrated, and without pedal oedema or peripheral lymphadenopathy. She weighed 88kg, her height was 1.6 metres, and her body mass index was $34.3 kg/m^2$, indicating Grade 1 obesity. Her waist circumference was 91cm, and her hip circumference was 102 cm, thereby giving a waist-to-hip ratio of 0.89, indicative of obesity. Her pulse was 92 beats per minute with a regular rhythm, normal volume, and in synchrony with other peripheral pulses. There was no thickening of the arterial wall. Her blood pressure was 220/120mmHg. The apex beat was at the fifth left intercostal space, on the mid-clavicular line. Her neck veins were not distended, and the jugular venous pressure was not raised. On auscultation of the heart, the first and second heart sounds were only heard, and there was no murmur.

Her respiratory rate was 20 cycles per minute; she had good air entry in her lung fields and vesicular breath sounds. Her visual acuity was 6/6 in both eyes. The vision was preserved in all eye fields. There was no swelling of the eyes or eyelids and no redness of the conjunctivae. The right and left corneas were transparent, there was normal depth of the anterior chambers and both pupils were symmetrical and reactive to light. There were normal red reflexes in both eyes, and the retina was normal. There was no evidence of arterio-venous thickening or the presence of exudates. Examination of the other systems was essentially normal.

A diagnosis of Severe Hypertension was made.

Management:

The patient's diagnosis and management plan was fully explained to her. She was admitted into the observation ward to afford her a period of rest and to commence antihypertensive drugs with the aim of reducing the raised blood pressure. She was given oral stat doses of tablets Nifedipine 20mg, Normoretic (Amiloride hydrochloride/ Hydrochlorothiazide) 5/50mg and Bromazepam (Lexotan) 1.5mg.

Six hours later, her blood pressure was 200/110mmHg. Although she was admitted for 24 hours, she refused an overnight stay in the ward because her husband was out of town, and she had no housekeeper to look after her children. She was placed on tablets of Amlodipine 10mg once daily, 1 tablet of Normoretic (5/50mg) daily, and tablets of Bromazepam 1.5mg nocte all for one week. Furthermore, she was asked to do an electrocardiogram and carry out laboratory investigations, which included urine analysis, fasting blood glucose, electrolytes, urea and creatinine assay, and fasting lipid profile. The patient was given a one-week follow-up appointment date.

One-week follow-up:

She attended the clinic for her follow-up visit, having the results of her investigations. She had missed two doses of Amlodipine tablets, ascribing the reason to financial limitations, including her husband's inability to provide finances, thereby leaving the burden on her. So, she did not buy a sufficient supply of her medications because she had to ration her available funds to take care of her children's needs, her laboratory investigations, and drugs. Her blood pressure on presentation was 150/100 mmHg. All the investigation results were normal.

At this visit, it was emphasized that drug use for her was for life. She was thus encouraged to use her registration in the National Health Insurance Scheme to offset the cost of drugs and reduce her financial burden instead of relying on out-of-pocket expenditures. She was encouraged to adopt the Dietary Approaches to Stop Hypertension (DASH) plan. These included eating more fruits, vegetables, and low-fat dairy foods; decreasing intake of foods that are high in saturated fat, cholesterol, and trans fats; higher intake of more whole-grain foods, fish, poultry, and nuts; and limiting sodium (salt), sweets, sugary drinks and red meats in her diet. She was also counseled on other lifestyle modifications like weight loss, exercise, and reduced alcohol consumption. Furthermore, the patient was counseled on contraception and the various available methods.

The advantages of good family planning, including health, social, and economic benefits, were explained to her, and the methods demonstrated using both visual and manual aids. She admitted that though she had heard about it, no one had ever explained it so clearly to her, possibly since she gave birth to all her children in the church. She was given a 2-week follow-up appointment, and it was requested that her husband accompany her on the visit.

Two weeks follow-up:

The patient was accompanied by her husband on this visit. Here, the importance of adherence to therapy and the role of the husband in achieving good adherence were discussed. Family planning measures were also discussed, and the importance of partner support was emphasized. Her husband agreed that she needed to be in optimal health to live a fruitful life and asserted his support for everything that would be required to achieve it. When asked about his financial state, he explained that he was now a registered cocoa farmer and would soon start receiving income from the sales of his crops. They had discussed and agreed that an intrauterine contraceptive device (IUCD) was the most suitable contraceptive method for them. They were asked to return to the clinic in a month for follow-up.

One-month follow-up:

She was reviewed a month following her previous visit. Her blood pressure was 135/80 mmHg, weight 86kg, and BMI 31.6kg/m^2. The headaches were gone, and she slept better at night. She had cut down significantly on carbohydrate staple foods in her meals and ate more fruits and vegetables. As regards contraception, an intrauterine contraceptive device had been inserted for her at a primary health center located near her home. She also stated that her husband was now providing money for the household as well as her drugs, which she was buying at an affordable rate through the National Health Insurance Scheme. This had greatly reduced the financial and mental stress she had been having. She was placed on monthly follow-up, and care is ongoing.

Summary:

A 44-year-old ward assistant was diagnosed with Severe Hypertension due to poor medication adherence. The financial barrier was a major factor contributing to her poor medication adherence. She was managed with drugs, health education on good adherence to therapy, and enlightenment on access to government health insurance.

Discussion:

Hypertension (HTN) or high blood pressure is defined as systolic blood pressure measurement of greater than or equal to 140mmHg or diastolic blood pressure greater than or equal to 90mmHg.[1,2]

It is a chronic disease of great magnitude, as an estimated 970 million people worldwide have the disease.[2] It is a leading cause of morbidity and mortality in Nigeria, as a meta-analysis done in Nigeria showed an overall prevalence of 28.9%.[3]

The achievement of therapeutic goals in hypertension can be done using pharmacological and non-pharmacological methods.[2,4] Non-pharmacological therapy involves appropriate lifestyle modifications aimed at lowering blood pressure, such as Dietary Approaches To Stop Hypertension (DASH), while pharmacological methods involve the use of medications such as calcium channel blockers, thiazide diuretics, angiotensin converting enzyme inhibitors, and angiotensin II receptor blockers as noted in the updated JNC-8 guidelines.[2,5] A drug combination of thiazide-type diuretics and calcium channel blockers as recommended in the JNC-8 guideline's recommendation for the black population, in addition to lifestyle counseling was used in the management of the index patient.

Adherence is defined as the extent to which a person's behavior – taking medication, following a diet, and/or executing lifestyle changes – corresponds with agreed recommendations from a health care provider.[6] Globally, the prevalence of chronic diseases is increasing; however, adherence to treatment regimens is persistently low.[7] Studies in developed countries show that only about 50% of all patients treat their chronic disease according to instructions.[8] Adherence has been recognized as a major factor in achieving optimal clinical outcomes in the management of chronic diseases like hypertension.[7] The index patient was a 44-year old hypertensive patient who was not adherent to her antihypertensive medication, which resulted in a negative clinical outcome.

Barriers to medication adherence have been grouped into categories, and they are patient-related factors such as cognitive impairment and co-morbidities; therapy-related factors.

It includes adverse events, dosing patterns, polypharmacy, treatment length, and routes of administration; healthcare system-related factors; and socio-economic related factors like treatment cost and financial support.[8,9] Financial hardship was the major barrier to this patient's medication adherence. It greatly limited her ability to purchase her drugs. Financial problems and treatment costs are among the important challenges facing patients living with hypertension.[8,9] Being a chronic illness, economic issues can significantly affect patient adherence to the extent that it leads to changes in the patient's medication plan and/or the permanent discontinuation of medication.[9]

Due to financial issues, this patient stopped taking her medications and resorted to using herbal remedies. Useful interventions that were applied by the family physician in her case included changing her drugs to cheaper yet effective alternatives and ensuring that the patient got enrolled in the health insurance scheme. These measures helped to improve medication adherence and management outcome.

This case served to highlight the role of healthcare financing as a factor in good medication adherence. The sources of revenues for healthcare can be public or private.[10] Public sources include government taxes, budget reallocation, donor schemes, debt relief, national health services like the National Health Insurance Scheme, social health insurance, private or voluntary health insurance, and community-based insurance. Private sources are mainly from out-of-pocket payments.[10] A large proportion of patients accessing healthcare in low-income countries use out-of-pocket payment methods, and this leads to difficulty in accessing healthcare services, including medications, as well as the risk of impoverishment due to catastrophic health expenses.[10]

Health education further played a critical role in enhancing the index patient's adherence to therapy. Studies have shown that better adherence to hypertensive medications is associated with the level of health education provided to patients.[10]

Hypertensive patients have a high risk of developing complications like cardiovascular diseases and kidney failure, which carry significant morbidity and mortality.[2] This patient was counseled on the dangers of developing these conditions, which would lead to even greater financial costs as well as disability.

Lesson learned/Recommendations:

To achieve drug adherence in patients with chronic illnesses like hypertension, health education within a patient-centered context is greatly emphasized.

References

1. Lim SS, Vos T, Flaxman AD, Danaei G, Shibuya K, Adair-Rohani H, *et al.* A comparative risk assessment of burden of disease and injury attributable to 67 risk factors and risk factor clusters in 21 regions, 1990-2010: A systematic analysis for the Global Burden of Disease Study 2010. Lancet 2012; 380:2224-60.

2. Bell K, Twiggs J, Olin BR. Hypertension: The silent killer: updated JNC-8 guideline recommendations. Alabama Pharmacy Association 2015. Summer 2015: continuing education. Available from: www.aparx.org

3. Adeloye D, Basquill C, Aderemi AV, Thompson JY, Obi FA. An estimate of the prevalence of hypertension in Nigeria: a systematic review and meta-analysis. Journal of Hypertension 2015; 33(2): 230-242

4. James PA, Oparil S, Carter BL, Cushman WC, Dennison-Himmelfarb C, Handler J et al. 2014 evidence-based guideline for the management of high

blood pressure in adults: report from the panel members appointed to the Eighth Joint National Committee (JNC 8). JAMA 2014; 311(5): 507 – 520.

5. Najimi A, Mostafavi F, Sharifirad G, Golshiri P. Barriers to medication adherence in patients with hypertension: A qualitative study. *J Educ Health Promot.* 2018; 7:24.

6. Brown MT, Bussell JK. Medication adherence: WHO cares? Mayo Clin Proc 2011; 86:304–14

7. Adeoye AM, Adebiyi AO, Adebayo OM, Owolabi MO. Medication adherence and 24-h blood pressure in apparently uncontrolled hypertensive Nigerian patients. Niger Postgrad Med J 2019: 26: 18-24

8. Oluwole EO, Osibogun O, Adegoke O, Adejimi AA, Adewole AM, Osibogun A. Medication adherence and patient satisfaction among hypertensive patients attending outpatient clinic in Lagos University

Teaching Hospital, Nigeria. Niger Postgrad Med J. 2019: 26: 129-37

9. Ibrahim OA, Olaniyan FA, Sule AG, Ibrahim BY. Socio-demographic and clinical factors affecting adherence to antihypertensive medications and blood pressure control among patients attending the family practice clinic in a tertiary hospital in northern Nigeria. Nigerian Journal of Family Practice. 2018; 9(1).

10. Osborn CY, Kripalani S, Goggins KM, Wallston KA. Financial strain is associated with medication non-adherence and worse self-rated health among cardiovascular patients. J Health Care Poor Underserved. 2017; 28 (1):499–513.

Chapter Eleven

Urinary Tract Infection In A 33-Year-Old Woman With An Ectopic Kidney

A 33-year-old housewife visited the clinic with complaints of fever, abdominal pain, and pain on passing urine of 1 week duration.

She was apparently well until a week before the presentation when she developed a fever that was high-grade, intermittent, and associated with chills and rigors. There was no history of yellowness of the eyes, cough, chest pain, or frequent stooling. She had abdominal pain, which was located at the lower part of the abdomen, intermittent, non-radiating, not associated with meals, and mildly relieved by rest. There was no history of vomiting, abnormal vaginal discharge, or abnormal vaginal bleeding.

She had no history of sexually transmitted infection, and her husband did not have a urethral discharge. Soon after, she developed a burning sensation whenever she passed urine. Her urine was whitish and reduced in quantity. There was increased frequency and urgency. She urinated about six to eight times daily as opposed to two to three times daily previously. There was no history of hematuria, incontinence, excessive thirst, excessive drinking or weight loss. She initially thought she had malaria, and so commenced and completed antimalarial drugs as well as Paracetamol and multivitamins. She also took enemas of herbal plants frequently while symptoms persisted. She had experienced similar symptoms in the past, which had been treated using over-the-counter medications; however, she decided to seek expert care when her abdominal pain persisted. The patient felt that her illness was due to a serious toilet infection and was afraid that she would be admitted. She had been unable to perform her daily chores and care for her young children, who could not yet fend for themselves. She expected that she would be treated adequately without the need for admission.

Her past medical and surgical history indicated she was not a known hypertensive, diabetic, asthmatic or sickle cell patient. She had a history of previous surgeries and blood transfusions. She was not on any routine drugs and was not allergic to any drugs. She attained menarche at the age of 12 years, her menstrual flow lasted between 4 – 5 days, and her menstrual cycle usually lasted 29 days. She used combined oral contraceptive pills for contraception. The patient was a Para 4^{+0} woman, all alive. She had undergone two Caesarean operations with no complications.

Her family and social history showed that the patient was the first child in a family of six children. All family members were alive and well. She was a housewife, married to a 46-year-old bulk provision trader. The family lived in a rented three-bedroom house with in-built toilet facilities and drank borehole water. She took alcoholic drinks occasionally and did not take tobacco in any form. Their source of healthcare financing was out of pocket. The family was at the school-age stage (Evelyn Duvall's family staging). Assessment of the family APGAR score was seven out of ten, depicting a functional family.

Her physical examination showed the patient was ill-looking and febrile with a temperature of 37.9 C. She was mildly dehydrated. There was no pallor, icterus, cyanosis, or bilateral pedal oedema. Her abdomen was mildly enlarged, soft, and moved with respiration. She had a Pfannenstiel incision scar. There was tenderness at the suprapubic region. There was no renal angle tenderness and no organ enlargement. Bowel sounds were normal and active. The pelvic examination showed a normal vulva and vagina with no vaginal discharge, masses, erosions, cysts, or lacerations. The cervix was soft and there was no tenderness on cervical motion. There was also no adnexal tenderness.

She was conscious and well-oriented. There was no sign of meningeal irritation or cranial nerve deficit. Her motor and sensory systems were normal. She had a pulse rate of 90 beats per minute, with a regular rhythm and normal volume. Her blood pressure was 130/80 mmHg. The first and second heart sounds were only heard. Her respiratory rate was 22 cycles per minute. There was equal chest expansion, resonant percussion notes, and vesicular breath sounds.

A diagnosis of Urinary tract infection (UTI), possibly cystitis, was made with a differential diagnosis of renal stones.

Management:

The diagnosis and management plan were explained to the patient. The laboratory investigations requested included complete blood count, urine analysis, fasting plasma glucose, urine microscopy, culture and sensitivity, and abdominopelvic ultrasound scan.

She was commenced on tablets of Paracetamol 1000 mg thrice daily for three days and tablets of Vitamin C 200mg daily for one week. She was advised to drink large quantities of water (about six to eight glasses daily), urinate anytime she felt the urge, observe good toilet hygiene and desist from sexual intercourse during the period of treatment. She was given a three-day appointment.

First follow up visit:

When she was seen three days later, she was in the company of her husband and pastor. She was very anxious. Her investigation results showed packed cell volume of 35%, total white cell count $10.6 \times 10^9/l$, with differential count of neutrophils 64%, eosinophils 1%, lymphocytes 35%; and erythrocyte sedimentation rate of 16 mm/hour by

Westergren method. Urine analysis results showed cloudy urine, very heavy protein, and epithelial cells. Fasting blood glucose was 4.8 mmol/l (3.5 – 5.5 mmol/l), and urine culture showed heavy growth of coliform organisms ($>10^2$/ml) after 72 hours. Abdomino-pelvic ultrasound scan showed the right kidney in its normal position with dimensions within normal limits. There was no evidence of renal calculi. The left renal bed was empty.

The patient disclosed that she had been told by the sonographer that she had only one kidney. Following this, she consulted friends that informed her that there were many reports of doctors who harvested patients' kidneys during surgery with general anesthesia, and there was a possibility that it had happened to her. She suspected that her kidney had been removed during one of her Caesarean operations, and she intended to seek legal action against the doctor who performed the surgery. Following her outburst, the managing physician tried to allay her anxiety by informing her that everything would be done to address her issues. She was asked to suspend legal action until all the relevant medical investigations had been done to ascertain her allegations. She was educated on the possibility of being born with a congenital abnormality of the kidneys. She was further requested to carry out intravenous urography as well as electrolytes, urea, and creatinine assay. She was commenced on tablets Cefuroxime (Zinnat) 500 mg twice daily for one week. They were asked to return for follow-up in a week.

2nd Follow-Up Visit:

The patient visited the clinic about three weeks later in the company of her husband. She stated that she did not honor her scheduled appointment because she was unhappy about her health issues. She was worried that having only one kidney would lead to her early death, and her children, being so young, would not have good maternal care. She now felt that an evil person had spiritually removed her kidney, and the matter had to be handled spiritually. The results of electrolytes, urea, and creatinine assay showed normal parameters and intravenous urogram revealed that the left kidney was located at the level of L4 L5, and S1 vertebrae, slightly to the left of the midline. The right kidney was normal in site, size, and function. No calculus or hydronephrosis were present. Both ureters and the urinary bladder were normal. All the findings were carefully explained to the patient. She was told that both kidneys were present however, one kidney was not found in its rightful place, and the condition would not lead to her early death. She was advised that since the condition was asymptomatic, no treatment was required, but she would need to have follow-up ultrasounds at regular intervals to detect any potential complications. She was educated on the importance of healthy nutrition, avoidance of alcohol and tobacco, adequate consumption of water, and regular medical check-ups. Following this, she still desired a second medical opinion, and so she was referred to a nephrologist.

The nephrologist gave similar advice to what she received in the family medicine clinic after which she returned to the family medicine clinic. Thereafter, she was less anxious about any potential health challenges consequent to her kidney abnormality. She expressed her willingness to cooperate with her management. The patient's care is currently receiving follow-up care at the general outpatient clinic.

Summary:

This was a 33-year-old woman diagnosed with a urinary tract infection. She had an incidental finding of left renal ectopia, which left her in great anxiety. She was treated for her urinary tract infection and properly counselled, using evidence of appropriate laboratory tests, about her congenital abnormality.

Discussion:

Urinary tract infection is the presence and growth of microorganisms in the organs that collect, store, and excrete urine in the body.[1] These organs include the bladder, ureters, and kidneys. The patient was a 33-year-old woman who presented with features of a urinary tract infection that had been recurrent. Statistics show that about 60% of all women and 12% of men have had it in their lifetime.[2] The infection has been reported to cause more than 8.1 million visits to healthcare providers each year.[2] Urinary tract infection is caused by *Escherichia coli* in 75-90% of cases.[3,4] Other causative organisms include *Staphylococcus saprophyticus, klebsiella species,* and *proteus mirabilis.*[3,4] In this patient, the causative organism found in her urine was Escherichia coli.

The disease could present clinically with dysuria, urinary frequency, cloudy or foul-smelling urine, lower abdominal pain, and hematuria or pyuria. This patient presented with urinary frequency, lower abdominal pain, and dysuria, which suggested she had cystitis. Renal calculi were a differential diagnosis in this patient because of similar symptoms of dysuria. However, it was excluded due to the absence of flank pain. In addition, the ultrasound result showed an absence of calculi in the kidneys. The risk factors include female gender, age (>34 years), frequent or recent sexual activity, pregnancy, diabetes mellitus, previous episodes of urinary tract infection, debility, poor perineal hygiene, estrogen deficiency, bladder outlet obstruction and congenital abnormalities of the kidneys such as ectopic kidney.[4,5]

An ectopic kidney, also known as renal ectopia, is a birth defect characterized by the abnormal location of one or both kidneys. [6]Abnormal locations could be the pelvis, inguinal or thoracic regions. It is a rare developmental anomaly occurring in 1 in 1000 births.[6] The pathology is usually a result of the arrested migration of one or both kidneys during the cephalic migration of the kidneys to their normal retroperitoneal location.[7] In most cases, patients are usually asymptomatic, with only about 1 in 10,000 cases ever being clinically recognized.[7] However, malposition of the ureters predisposes them to ureteral obstruction, calculi, and recurrent urinary tract infection.[6,7] This woman's kidney was located in the midline and not in the correct position, which is the renal groove. She had a history of similar recurrent symptoms, thus showing that the renal anomaly was a major risk factor in her illness.

Due to the rarity of the condition as well as its vague atypical symptoms, the diagnosis is usually an incidental finding during radiological evaluations of the genitourinary system.[6] In this particular patient, it was an incidental radiological finding. Incidental discovery of a congenital abnormality in an adult may lead to psychosocial symptoms in a patient like fear and false illness perceptions,[8,9] as was seen in the index patient. An inquiry into the ideas that patients have about their illness can address these perceptions. This patient believed that her kidney had been wrongfully removed and she was spiritually attacked. These perceptions were corrected by properly health-educating her.

The diagnosis of UTI can be done through urine analysis or urine culture using a mid-stream urine specimen. Urine culture is the gold standard as it confirms the presence of bacteriuria and the antimicrobial susceptibility of the infecting pathogen.[2,3] Both investigations were done on this patient. More investigations can be done to exclude other differential diagnoses. Treatment is usually done with antibiotics.[10] The patient was treated with Cefuroxime, a third-generation cephalosporin because she gave a history of recurrence and frequent use of over-the-counter drugs, which might have led to resistance. She had a good treatment outcome with the drug.

Lessons Learned/ Recommendations:

Congenital malformations are rare events that have significant impacts on individuals, families, health-care systems, and societies. It is recommended that there should be more advocacy for the prevention of preventable anomalies through vaccination, adequate intake of folic acid or iodine through fortification of staple foods, as well as adequate antenatal care.

References

1. Hooton TM. Uncomplicated urinary tract infection. N Engl J Med. 2012; 366:1028-1037

2. Iregbu K, Nwajiobi-princewill P. Urinary tract infections in a tertiary hospital in Abuja, Nigeria. Afr J Cln Exper Microbiol. 2013;14(3): 169-73

3. Oluwafemi TT, Akinbodewa AA, Ogunleye A, Adejumo OA. Urinary tract infections and antibiotic sensitivity pattern of uropathogens in a tertiary hospital in Southwest Nigeria. Sahel Med J. 2018; 21:18-22

4. Glover M, Moreira CG, Sperandio V, Zimmern P. Recurrent urinary tract infections in healthy and non-pregnant women. Urological Science. 2014;25(1):1-8

5. Oladeinde BH, Omoregie R, Olley M, Anunibe JA. Urinary tract infection in a rural community of Nigeria. *N Am J Med Sci* 2011; 3:75-7.

6. Lema VM. Sexual activity and the risk of acute uncomplicated urinary tract infection in premenopausal

women: implications for reproductive health programming. Obstetrics and Gynecology International Journal. 2018; 9:1

7. Ilah BG, Sakajiki AM, Aghadueki S, Bassey E, Kolawole T, Adeniji AO. Ectopic pelvic kidney in a neonate in Gusau, Zamfara, Northwestern Nigeria. Sahel Med J 2015; 18: 89-90

8. Lu C, Tain Y, Yeung K, Tiao M. Case report of ectopic pelvic kidney with urinary tract infection presenting as lower abdominal pain in a child. Pediatrics and Neonatology. 2011; 52(2):117-120

9. Majoor BCJ, Andela CD, Quispel CR, Rotman M, Dijkstra PDS, Hamdy NAT et al. Illness perceptions are associated with quality of life in patients with fibrous dysplasia. *Calcif Tissue Int*. 2018; 02(1):23–31

10. Juergens MC, Seekatz B, Moosdorf RG, Petrie KJ, Rief W. Illness beliefs before cardiac surgery predict

disability, quality of life, and depression 3 months later. *J. Psychosom. Res.* 2010; 68:553–560

Chapter Twelve

Food Poisoning In A Nurse

The patient, a 36-year-old nurse, presented at the outpatient clinic with abdominal pain, frequent stooling, and vomiting of 3 days' duration.

She was apparently well until three days before the presentation, when she developed abdominal pain. The pain was colicky, continuous, and sharp. It was relieved by walking around and aggravated by ingestion of food or drinks. A few hours after the onset of pain, she started stooling. Stooling occurred about eleven times within two days. Stools were watery and contained mucus. She also observed blood during one episode of stooling. In three days, she had experienced about eight episodes of vomiting; vomitus contained previously ingested food and fluids. There was associated fever, headache and generalized weakness. She had no urinary symptoms or yellowness of the eyes.

About six hours before the onset of these symptoms, the patient and two friends had joined a commercial bus to travel to another town. While they sat in the bus and waited to start their journey, they bought and ate grilled peppered snails sold by a food vendor that hawked food to passengers in the bus that they were travelling in. The food had a slightly spoiled taste. Her friends had called her to complain of similar symptoms, and one of them had even been admitted to a private clinic. Since the onset of symptoms, she had ingested some tablets of Tetracycline and oral rehydration salt solution, but she had no relief. She decided to visit the clinic because she saw blood in her stool. She felt that the symptoms were due to the snails she had eaten. She had missed going to work for two days because of her illness. She was afraid that she appeared to be getting worse even after having taken drugs, and she expected to be treated for the illness.

Her past medical and surgical history showed she had no history of hypertension, epilepsy, asthma, diabetes or sickle cell disease. There was no history of previous surgeries or blood transfusions.

She was Para 2^{+0}. Her menarche had commenced at 11 years; she had a regular 28-day cycle and a menstrual flow of 4 days. She used an intrauterine device for contraception.

She was the fifth child in a family of 6 children, 4 females and 2 males. Both parents were alive. She was a senior nursing officer at a tertiary hospital and was happily married to a 40-year-old naval officer. They had 2 children, one male and one female, who were in secondary school. The family lived in a rented 3-bedroom house. They drank borehole water and used water cistern toilets. Assessment of family Apgar was 10 out of 10. Their source of health financing was through the national health insurance scheme.

A physical examination revealed an acutely ill woman who was febrile with a temperature of 38.3^{0}C, mildly pale, and dehydrated. There was no jaundice, cyanosis, peripheral lymphadenopathy, or pedal oedema. Abdominal examination showed her abdomen was flat and moved with respiration. There was generalized tenderness. Guarding and rebound tenderness were absent. The spleen and liver were not enlarged. The kidneys were not ballotable. The bowel sounds were hyperactive. She was conscious and well-oriented. There was no sign of meningeal irritation or cranial nerve deficit. Her motor and sensory systems were normal.

Her pulse rate was 98 beats per minute. The pulse had a regular rhythm and moderate volume. Her blood pressure was 100/70 mmHg. Her jugular venous pressure was not raised; the apex beat was at the fifth left intercostal space, mid-clavicular line. Her first and second heart sounds were only heard. There was no murmur.

A diagnosis of Food poisoning was made.

Management:

The diagnosis and management plan were explained to the patient, including the need for admission, and she consented. She was admitted to the observation ward of the outpatient clinic. The laboratory investigations carried out included complete blood count, stool microscopy, and culture as well as blood film for malaria parasites. The results showed no malaria parasites on the blood film, haemoglobin estimation of 12.1 g/dl, packed cell volume 36%, white cell count 9.8 $\times 10^9$/l with a differential count of 68% neutrophils, 31% lymphocytes, and 1% eosinophil. *Escherichia coli* was isolated on stool culture.

She was commenced on one liter of intravenous normal saline infusion 6 hourly for 12 hours, intramuscular

Promethazine 25 mg stat, intravenous Ciprofloxacin 200mg stat to be followed by tablets Ciprofloxacin 500mg 12 hourly for 5 days, intravenous Metronidazole 500mg stat to be followed by tablets Metronidazole 400 mg 8 hourly for 5 days, tablets Loperamide 4 mg stat followed by tablets Loperamide 2 mg per loose stool. She was also given tablets of Hyoscine butyl bromide (Buscopan) 20mg twice daily for 3 days.

On admission:

She was reviewed at six and twelve hours after admission. She had an episode of stooling, which did not contain blood while on admission, but there was no vomiting or abdominal pain. Her vital signs showed a temperature of 37.5^0C, pulse rate of 86 beats per minute, and blood pressure of 110/70 mmHg. She was told to take generous amounts of fluids, including oral rehydration solution, and to complete her oral medications. She was discharged from the Observation ward and given a three-day appointment. Before discharge, she was counseled on the importance of food hygiene, the dangers of eating street-vendor food, the importance of hand washing as well as proper food storage for the prevention of food-borne diseases.

Follow-up visit:

At her follow-up visit three days later, she had no complaints. Physical examination showed normal findings. The patient was subsequently discharged from follow-up.

Summary:

A 36-year-old nurse with a history of abdominal pain, bloody stool, and vomiting, which began some hours after her consumption of street-vended snails. Management involved fluid and antibiotic therapy in addition to health education on food hygiene.

Discussion:

Food poisoning is an acute intestinal disease acquired by ingestion of food or drinks contaminated by toxic agents. These toxic agents could be microorganisms such as bacteria, viruses, and fungi; parasites such as intestinal worms, toxins, and heavy metals like lead and mercury.[1,2] The symptoms may include diarrhoea, vomiting and abdominal pain.[3] In severe cases, there could be bloody stools, high fever, and shock due to dehydration. The patient presented with abdominal pain, frequent stooling with blood in stool, and vomiting, which were typical symptoms of food poisoning. Symptoms can last between 1 and 10 days and may be mild or severe enough to require hospitalization. The index patient was hospitalized for this illness. Her two travel companions who ate the same food also developed similar symptoms.

Bacterial agents involved in food poisoning include *Staphylococcus aureus, Bacillus cereus, Clostridium botulinum, Vibrio cholera, Salmonella typhimurium,*

Escherichia coli, and *Shigella* species.[3,4] Viral agents implicated in the etiology include Norovirus. The incubation periods for etiological agents vary, with *Staph aureus* having an incubation period of 1-6 hours, *S. typhi* 12 – 72 hours, Norovirus 12 – 48 hours, *C. botulinum* 18 – 36 hours and *V. cholera* 1 – 4 days.[5,6] In the index patient, *Escherichia coli* was the etiological agent isolated on stool culture.

The diagnosis involves isolating the causative organisms on stool microscopy.[6,7] However, the absence of microorganisms does not rule out the diagnosis.[6,7] In staphylococcal food poisoning, the symptoms are primarily due to enterotoxins produced by Staphylococcus. So, the disease is more a case of intoxication than an infection. Treatment involves symptom management as well as eradicating the offending organism.[2,4] Rehydration using intravenous fluids and drinking is necessary to prevent dehydration and shock.[4] These treatment modalities were used in the management of this patient.

Some risk factors in the occurrence of food poisoning include age, gender, socioeconomic status, place of residence, health status, and poverty.[7,8] Poverty enhances food safety problems through low levels of literacy, poor knowledge in food handling, unsanitary living conditions, lack of access to clean water, and unhygienic transportation and food storage.[6, 8] In Nigeria, the entire culture of food handling, preparation and storage is generally below acceptable standards.[9] Many local practices also do not enhance food hygiene. A large proportion of food outlets that cater to people of low socio-economic class are situated in dirty, unhygienic environments,[7,9,] and it is not uncommon to also find middle-class people patronizing these outlets. The index patient was a senior nursing officer with a considerable number of years in health practice, yet that did not restrain her from buying food being sold by the roadside, thus showing the poor food safety culture found among people in developing countries.

Prevention modalities for food poisoning should focus on the method and environment of food preparation, sanitary conditions, and food inspection policies.[10] This patient developed food poisoning only a few hours after ingesting contaminated food, and this strongly signified the poor hygienic state of the method of food preparation and environment.

Lessons Learned/ Recommendations:

The food safety policies and implementation in Nigeria are very inadequate. There should be an evaluation of policies regarding food safety in the community, and family physicians play an integral role in advocacy on this issue. The culture of street vending, as well as patronage of food sold on the streets, should be discouraged. There should be increased awareness of preventive measures like handwashing and proper disposal of waste.

References

1. Kasule M, Malangu N. Profile of acute poisoning in three health districts of Botswana. African Journal of Primary Health Care and Primary Medicine. 2009; 1:1
2. Weiler N, Leotta GA, Zarate MN. Foodborne outbreak associated with ultra-pasteurized milk in the Republic of Paraguay. Revista Argentina de Microbiologia. 2011; 43(1): 33-36
3. Fatiregun AA, Oyebade OA, Oladokun L. Investigation of an outbreak of food poisoning. Tropical Journal of Health Sciences. 2010; 17:1
4. Scallan E, Hoekstra RM, Angulo FJ, Tauxe RV, Widdowson M, Roy SL et al. Foodborne illness acquired in the United States – major pathogens. Emerging Infectious Diseases. 2011; 17:1
5. Painter JA, Hoekstra RM, Ayers T, Tauxe RV, Braden CR, Angulo JA et al. Attribution of foodborne illnesses, hospitalizations, and deaths to food commodities by

using outbreak data, United States, 1998–2008. *Emerging Infectious Diseases.* 2013;19 (3):407-415. doi:10.3201/eid1903.111866.

6. Fashae K, Ogunsola F, Aarestrup FM. Antimicrobial susceptibility and serovars of Salmonella from chickens and humans in Ibadan, Nigeria. The Journal of Infection in Developing Countries. 2010; 4:8. 484-494

7. Akhtar S, Sarker MR, Hossain A. Microbiological food safety: a dilemma of developing societies. Critical Reviews in Microbiology. 2014; 40(4): 348-359

8. Sasson A. Food security for Africa: an urgent global challenge. Agriculture and Food Security. 2012; 1(2): 1-16

9. Onyeneho SN, Hedberg CW. An assessment of food safety needs of restaurants in Owerri, Imo State, Nigeria. International Journal of Environmental Research and Public Health. 2013; 10(8): 3296-3309

10. Osagbemi G, Abdullahi A, Aderibigbe S. Knowledge, attitudes and practice concerning food poisoning among residents of Okene Metropolis, Nigeria. Research Journal of Social Sciences. 2010; 1(4): 61-64.

Chapter Thirteen

Vaso-Occlusive Crisis In A 7-Year-Old Sickler

A 7-year-old female patient was brought to the Children's Emergency Room with bone pain and a fever of 3 days' duration.

She was a known sickle cell disease patient who had been diagnosed three years earlier at a private hospital. About three days before her presentation at the hospital, she complained of pain in her legs and arms, which was insidious in onset. It gradually became so severe that she could not walk and screamed when her arms or legs were touched. There were no relieving factors, and the pain was aggravated by mobility. There was associated headache, loss of appetite, and abdominal pain, which was generalized and intermittent. She had two episodes of vomiting; vomitus was copious, bilious and contained ingested food. There was no history of constipation or diarrhea.

The fever was of sudden onset, high-grade, intermittent, and relieved with ingestion of Paracetamol tablets. There was no cough, ear pain or discharge, pain when urinating, convulsions or throat pain. Since the onset of the illness, she had been given Paracetamol tablets, Ibuprofen syrup and Zithromax syrup. There was no blurred vision, dizziness, fainting attacks, difficulty in breathing, chest pain or palpitations.

The patient's mother felt she was having a crisis which was triggered because of her playing in the rain a week earlier. She was afraid that this crisis would cause her death as it had progressed so rapidly in as short as three days. She had missed going to school, thereby missing her first school excursion. Her mother expected that she would be given drugs to restore her quickly to sound health to save her life.

In the past medical and surgical history, the patient had been admitted several times in the past two years for malaria and bone pain at different health facilities. She was not asthmatic, diabetic or epileptic. There was no history of previous surgeries or blood transfusions. She took Multivitamin syrup daily based on the advice of a chemist. She had no known allergy to any drugs.

Her pregnancy was not planned, as her parents were not intending to get married when it occurred. Her mother discovered her genotype was AS when she booked for antenatal care. She was admitted for antepartum hemorrhage during pregnancy. The patient was born at term through a Caesarean delivery at a hospital. The indication for Caesarean delivery was obstructed labor. Her birth weight was 3.7kg, and she cried at birth. Her developmental milestones were normal for her age.

Her immunization records showed that she had completed her immunization for age according to the National Program on Immunization in Nigeria. The patient was exclusively breastfed for 2 months before commencing on infant formula and semi-solid foods. She ate regular family meals.

The patient was a first-year pupil in a private elementary school. She was the first of two children; she had a younger brother who was two years old. Her father was a 33-year-old Mobile Police officer, while her mother was a 29-year-old food caterer. They lived in a two-bedroom apartment, drank borehole water and had mosquito nets on their windows, which were not insecticide-treated. Both parents had sickle cell trait with genotype AS. Her brother's genotype was AA. Her mother lamented that their home was full of conflicts because of the patient's recurrent ill-health. Although her mother knew her genotype, her father only discovered his genotype when the patient started having crises; initially, they did not understand the reason for her frequent ill-health until a laboratory test revealed her genotype. Her father blamed her mother for not informing him and marrying him despite her medical condition. The family was at the school age children family stage of Evelyn Duvall's model. The family APGAR score assessment (according to the mother) was 5/10 depicting a moderately dysfunctional family.

The general physical examination revealed an acutely ill girl in pain. She was febrile with a temperature of 39.2^0 C, moderately pale, icteric, and mildly dehydrated. There was no cyanosis, peripheral lymphadenopathy or pedal oedema. She was conscious, alert and irritable. There were no signs of meningeal irritation or cranial nerve deficit. Examination of the musculoskeletal system showed diffuse tenderness of the arms, forearms and legs. Further examination of this system was deferred because she was in severe distress. Her pulse rate was 110 beats per minute with a regular rhythm and full volume. Blood pressure was 100/60 mmHg. The apex beat was at the 5th left intercostal space on the mid- clavicular line. The first and second heart sounds were only heard.

The respiratory rate was 26 cycles per minute. She had normal chest expansion, resonant percussion notes and vesicular breath sounds. Abdominal examination showed the abdomen was enlarged, soft and moved with respiration. The liver was enlarged 8 cm below the right costal margin, non-tender and with a smooth surface. The spleen was not enlarged, and the kidneys were not ballotable. A diagnosis of Vaso-occlusive crisis in a known Sickler was made.

Management:

The patient was admitted and managed as an emergency. The investigations done for her were a complete blood count, blood film for malaria parasites, and urine analysis.

The results showed a packed cell volume of 26%, white blood cell count of 5.1 x 10⁹/l with a differential count of 60% neutrophil, 1% eosinophil and 39% lymphocyte. Ring forms of Plasmodium falciparum were seen in her blood film. The urine analysis showed parameters within normal limits.

1st day of admission:

She was commenced on intravenous fluid 5% Dextrose in half strength normal saline solution. The management plan was to rehydrate the patient with 150% maintenance fluid, pain management and treat of underlying triggers of the crisis. According to her weight, she was to receive a total of 2250 ml of fluid (fluid deficit plus maintenance) over 24 hours. The drip was set at 31 drops per minute to prevent over hydration. She also received intravenous Pentazocine 15mg 6 hourly for 24 hours, tablets of Acetaminophen 500mg eight hourly for 3 days and intramuscular β-

Arteether (Paluther) 3mg/kg (60mg) daily for 3 days. On completion of the β-Arteether injection, she would take tablets Artemether/lumefantrine 20/120 mg orally, one dose stat, then one dose 8 hours later the first day, to be followed by one dose twice daily for the remaining 2 days. The patient was sponged with tepid water, and her vital signs were monitored every 4 hours for the first 24 hours. After six hours of admission, bone pains were observed to have reduced, and she was able to sleep. Her temperature was 38.9^0C; her respiratory rate was 20 cycles per minute, and her pulse rate was 90 beats per minute. Liberal oral fluid intake was also encouraged as much as she could tolerate.

2nd – 3rd days of admission:

During this period, there were complaints of weakness by her mother, although bone pain had reduced appreciably. She had received oral fluids and semi-solid food (custard) and had tolerated them. Her temperature was 38.1^0C. Other vital signs were within normal limits. Pentazocine and other medications were continued. She later continued on 700ml of intravenous fluid 12 hourly for 24 hours.

4th day of admission:

There were no complaints of pain, fever, vomiting or other symptoms. Her temperature was 37.4^{0}C, pulse rate 88^{0}C and respiratory rate 16 cycles per minute. Examination of other systems showed normal findings. Subsequently, her parents were educated on the management of a child with sickle cell disease and factors which could precipitate crises. She was to drink enough water daily, avoid extremes of temperature, sleep under insecticide-treated nets always, and their surroundings fumigated and cleared of bushes as well as stagnant pools of water to prevent malaria. They were told that the possible risk factors for the crisis she had were malaria and cold weather. She commenced on routine medications, which were tablets of Paludrin 100mg daily orally, 1 tablet each of Folic Acid and Vitamin B-complex daily orally. Her parents were advised to discontinue multivitamin syrups or iron-containing formulations. Following this, the patient was discharged, and a one-week appointment was scheduled.

Follow-up:

She was seen one week later with her parents and there were no complaints about her health. The examination showed normal vital signs. PCV was done, and the result was 27%. On enquiry about the family's state, her mother stated that the illness had been tough on their home. She enquired about a permanent cure for sickle cell disease as certain friends had told her that there were herbal remedies for it. Her father also was deeply concerned about the patient's health as well as the financial and social strain it had on their family.

Health education on sickle cell disease was reiterated, and they were informed that there was no cure for the disease as it was an abnormality inherited through her parents; however, she could live a healthy life with the disease if there was medication adherence, good lifestyle modification with avoidance of factors precipitating crises, healthy nutrition and regular medical check-ups.

The parents were also given genetic counselling, counselling on risks in subsequent children, in-vitro tests during pregnancy, adoption and contraceptive advice.

A medical report was issued to the patient's school authorities to alert them of her health status, restrain her from school activities that could predispose her to crises and seek their cooperation in her management. Subsequently, she was given monthly appointments and placed on continued care.

Summary:

A 7-year-old sickle cell disease patient was brought to the Children's Emergency room in Vaso-occlusive crisis. Her condition was worsened by a dysfunctional home environment brought about by her health condition. Apart from medical management, parental counselling on home care of sickle cell patients was done.

Discussion:

Sickle cell disease is a genetic hemolytic anaemia due to abnormality in haemoglobin from a single glutamic acid to valine substitution at position 6 of the beta- globin polypeptide chain.[1,2] There is red blood cell deformation resulting in occlusion of blood vessels, local tissue hypoxia and damage.[1] It is inherited as an autosomal recessive trait. The index patient was a 7-year-old girl who inherited the disease from her parents, who were carriers, as an autosomal recessive trait.

Data from the World Health Organization has reported that globally, there are about 20-25 million people living with the disease, and of this number, about 15 million are found in sub-Saharan Africa.[1] In Nigeria, there is a high prevalence of the disease, as reports from WHO show that 24% of Nigerians carry the mutant gene, with approximately 150,000 hospital admissions per year from sickle cell disease.[1]

The clinical course of the disease is typically characterized by variable periods of steady states interrupted by crises.[1,3] The types of crises that could occur are Vaso-occlusive crises and acute anaemic crises. Vaso-occlusive crisis clinically manifests with bone pain involving the long bones. It could be acute, presenting with sudden onset of pain in the bones, or it could be chronic, such as in chronic osteomyelitis, septic arthritis and avascular necrosis of the femoral head. Acute anaemic crisis could be hyperhemolytic manifesting with anaemia and jaundice, sequestration manifesting with anaemia and splenomegaly or aplastic manifesting with fever and anaemia. The patient presented with severe bone pain, which was a pointer to the diagnosis of Vaso-occlusive crisis. A vaso-occlusive crisis may occur spontaneously or may be precipitated by infections, extremes in temperature, dehydration or stress. In the index patient, the likely precipitants of her crisis were exposure to cold and malaria infection.

Treatment of Vaso-occlusive crisis can be achieved with analgesics like acetaminophen, non-steroidal anti-inflammatory drugs, opioids and cytotoxic drugs like Hydroxyurea, depending on pain severity. Other pain management strategies include heat pads, physiotherapy, acupuncture and transcutaneous electrical nerve stimulation. Adjuvant therapy includes intravenous fluids for adequate hydration, sedatives and anxiolytics for relief of anxiety, anticonvulsants and laxatives. In this patient, opioids were prescribed because pain severity was so high that even touch caused pain, and she was adequately hydrated with intravenous fluids. Subsequently, routine hematinic (Folic acid and vitamin B complex) and malaria prophylaxis (Paludrin) were prescribed for chronic administration.

Sickle cell disease has been found to have an impact on the family dynamics of affected families.[7] It can cause family dysfunction, and likewise, family dysfunction can aggravate the disease. Family challenges could be a financial burden, neglect of other family members, frequent school and work absenteeism, and cultural and religious misperceptions.[7,8] Adequate health education could produce positive health outcomes in patients and families. The index patient was in a dysfunctional family setting ridden with parental conflicts and poor information, which might explain the constant crises occurring multiple times yearly that she had suffered.

Lessons Learned/Recommendation:

The importance of pre-conception care in young, unmarried people cannot be overemphasized. It is recommended that family physicians give genetic counseling to patients, particularly unmarried ones, as part of general health education. Parents and caregivers of sicklers should be properly educated on the management for them to give adequate mental and psychosocial support to these sicklers.

References

1. Cheesman S. Sickle cell disease: symptoms, complications and management. Clinical Pharmacist. 2015; 7(8). online

2. Ademola SA. Management of sickle cell disease: a review for physician education in Nigeria (Sub-Saharan Africa). Anemia. 2015, Article ID 791498, 21 pages.

3. Makani J, Ofori-Acquah SF, Nnodu O, Wonkam A, Ohene-Frempong K. Sickle cell disease: new opportunities and challenges in Africa. The Scientific World Journal. 2013; Article ID 193252.

4. Mousa SA, Al Momen A, Al Sayegh F. Management of painful vaso- occlusive crisis of sickle-cell anemia: consensus opinion. Clin Appl Thromb Hemost. 2010; 16:365–376

5. Bolarinwa RA, Akinola NO, Aboderin OA, Durosinmi MA. The role of malaria in vaso-occlusive crisis of

adult patients with sickle cell disease. J Med Sci. 2010; 1:407–411

6. Ahmed SG. The role of infections in the pathogenesis of vaso-occlusive crisis in patients with sickle cell disease. Mediterr Haematol Infect Disease. 2011;3(1)

7. Olaniyi JA, Alagbe AE, Olutoogun TA, Busari OE. Multiple bone and joint diseases in a Nigerian with sickle cell anemia: a case report. Mediterr J Hematol Infect Dis. 2012; 4(1).

8. Adegoke SA, Kuteyi EA. The psychosocial burden of sickle cell disease on the family, Nigeria. Afr J Prim Health Care Fam Med. 2012; 4 (1):380.

9. Brown B, Okereke J, Lagunju I, Orimadegun A, Ohaeri J, Akinyinka O. Burden of healthcare of carers of children with sickle cell disease in Nigeria. Health Soc Care Community. 2010; 18:289–295.

10. Anie KA, Egunjobi FE, Akinyanju OO. Psychosocial impact of sickle cell disorder: Perspectives from a Nigerian setting. Global. Health. 2010; 6(2):1–6.

Chapter Fourteen

Scabies In A 13-Year-Old Student

A 13-year-old male student presented at the clinic with rashes on the groin and itching of five months' duration. The patient was apparently well until five months prior to presentation when he developed rashes on his groin. These rashes initially appeared at the inner part of both thighs and then spread to encompass the penis and scrotum. They were not painful but were very itchy, which made him scratch vigorously, thereby sustaining wounds on his skin. The itching was worse at night and anytime he felt hot or sweated.

There was a history of contact with people having similar complaints. His grandmother and four other children living in the same compound with them had the symptoms. There was a history of having had similar complaints about a year earlier when he was in boarding school. At that time, he had rashes on his wrists and between his fingers. His grandmother said the water used by the students for bathing in the school was the reason for the infection, as so many students had similar complaints. Due to this, he had been removed from the school to another one where he was a day student. For these complaints, he had used Sulphur cream, Nixoderm cream and Funbact-A cream to no avail. His grandmother was worried that the rashes might affect his fertility in the future and desired that he should be cured of it. The patient was also worried about the embarrassment the itching caused him in school among his classmates and hoped to have a permanent cure.

His past medical and surgical history indicated the patient had suffered a fracture of his left forearm when he was 9 years old and was treated using a Plaster of Paris cast. There was no history of chronic illness. The pregnancy, birth and developmental history showed that his pregnancy was planned and uneventful. He was born at term in a hospital. His birth weight was 3.9kg. His developmental milestones were normal for his age. His immunization history showed his immunization records were complete, as seen on his immunization card.

He was a third-year Junior Secondary School student and the only child of his parents. Both parents were law enforcement officers and were on transfer at the time of the hospital visit, so he lived with his paternal grandmother. She was a bulk trader in dry fish. His parents were married but had lived apart most of the time because of their jobs; however, his grandmother affirmed that they provided good financial support for them and visited frequently. The patient and his grandmother lived in a rented three-bedroom apartment in a complex having six apartments. His grandmother conducted her trade from home and because she was always at home, some children in the complex usually stayed in their home after school while waiting for their own parents to return from work.

A physical examination showed a healthy-looking boy who was not febrile, not pale, not jaundiced, and not dehydrated. There was significant peripheral lymphadenopathy. There were hyper-pigmented areas on his fingers and ventral parts of his wrists. Examination showed numerous skin lesions on the inner thighs, penis and scrotum. These lesions consisted of papules, nodules, vesicles, and some healed wounds. Examination of the urogenital system showed that both testes were present, and there was no abnormality of the phallus.

His pulse rate was 74 beats per minute, with the pulse having a regular rhythm and normal volume. His blood pressure was 100/70mmHg; jugular venous pressure was not raised, and the apex beat was at the fifth left intercostal space on the mid-clavicular line. The respiratory rate was 16 cycles per minute. Chest expansion was equal on both sides. He had vesicular breath sounds, and his chest was clinically clear. An abdominal examination revealed a flat abdomen that moved with respiration. There were no areas of tenderness and no organomegaly. The bowel sounds were normal and active. Examination of other systems did not show any abnormalities.

A diagnosis of Scabies with secondary bacterial infection was made.

Management:

The diagnosis was explained to the patient and his grandmother. They were told that the possible cause of the problem was skin infestation by a mite acquired through skin contact with another infected person. Laboratory investigations, which included VDRL test and HIV screening, were requested. He was given topical 5% Permethrin cream to be applied overnight (approximately 12 hours) and then washed off, capsules of Ampicillin-cloxacillin 500 mg six-hourly for 5 days, and tablets of Promethazine (Phenergan) 25 mg nocte for 5 nights. Permethrin was to be repeated after one week. The same medications were also prescribed for his grandmother. Furthermore, they were advised to wash all their clothes and bedding with hot water and spread them out in the sun. They were also told to spread their mattresses in the sun for about three days, bringing them into the house at night; however, they would not sleep on these mattresses during that time.

His grandmother was told to inform the parents of the other children who had the infection of the need for them to be treated to eradicate the infection and prevent its spread within the apartment complex. However, she suggested that it would be better for the physician to tell them and help educate them on health problems. That would convince them to purchase the drugs for the treatment of their children. He was given a two-week appointment. A home visit was also scheduled four days later, with the aim of carrying out health education and promotion for the members of the complex in which they lived.

Home visit:

The home visit took place four days after the previous clinic visit. The surroundings were generally tidy, with good waste disposal. The apartment where the patient and his grandmother lived had a tidy living room, but the bedrooms were cluttered with various items. Both the patient and his grandmother shared a room, sleeping on one mattress. The bedding was not clean and usually changed on two to three weekly occasions. Towels, bathing sponges, and other fomites were also shared between them. They were advised not to share personal items like towels, toothbrushes, and combs. They were advised to practice good hygiene within the home. A visit to their neighbors revealed that three adults and four children had scabies. A stat dose of oral tablets of Ivermectin 200µg/kg/dose was prescribed for them, and this was to be repeated after one week. They were also counseled on good hygiene.

Follow-up:

He was seen a week after the home visit with his grandmother. He admitted that the itching had ceased, and he was no longer uncomfortable. Most of the papules were drying off and presented as scabs on the body. All the investigation results were normal. He was asked to repeat the application of Permethrin overnight for 12 hours. His grandmother had also observed an improvement in her symptoms. On inquiry about the state of the neighbors' children, she stated that all the parents had complied with the health education, and the lesions had cleared from a large majority of them. She, however, had decided to restrict access for visitors into their bedrooms. Good hygiene was reiterated, and the patient was given a one-week appointment.

At the subsequent visit, the patient had no complaints. All lesions had cleared from his skin, and he was in a stable clinical state. He was thus discharged from follow-up.

Summary:

A 13-year-old secondary school student came to the clinic with groin rashes and itching and was diagnosed with Scabies. From him, the infection had spread to his grandmother and other children, thus prompting a home visit for health education and promotion.

Discussion:

Human scabies is a skin disease caused by infestation with a mite called Sarcoptes scabiei var hominis.[1] It is one of the most common dermatological conditions, accounting for a substantial proportion of skin disease in developing countries, and has been identified by the World Health

Organization (WHO) as one of the Neglected Tropical Diseases (NTDs).[2] It is estimated that about 200 million people are affected by this disease globally at any time, with an estimated average prevalence of 5 – 10% in children.[2,3] The burden of this disease was evident in the index case being presented, as the disease was found in as many as ten people within one living space.

Scabies are transmitted through direct and prolonged contact with an infected skin or rarely by using contaminated objects.[4] In school children, the disease often spreads rapidly because of their close contact as well as overcrowding within schools.[5] Overcrowding is an important factor in the spread of scabies, as it has been reported that closed communities and institutional facilities are likely to experience high endemic rates.[6] Hygiene is another factor that is linked to the transmission of scabies as poor hygiene can compound the problem of overcrowded living quarters.[6] All these factors are important as they can be utilized in community prevention of the disease. The index patient first acquired the infection when he was a boarding student in school, thus showing the likelihood of skin contact. In the current presentation, the infection spread from him to his grandmother and four other children who were usually near him.

Scabies presents with lesions commonly affecting the hands, wrists, ankles, and feet. Due to the mite's predilection for warm areas of the body, lesions could also be found at the elbows, underneath the breasts, and genital areas. Other clinical forms of scabies, such as crusted scabies (Norwegian scabies), exist. This form is present in severely ill or immune-compromised patients.[7] The index patient had skin lesions around his genitals and inner thighs, thus exhibiting the illness pathogenesis.

Diagnosis of scabies infestation is based mainly on clinical recognition of the typical features of infestation.[2] When necessary, diagnosis can be supported by the identification of mites in skin scrapings or through visual imaging techniques such as dermatoscopy, polymerase chain reaction, and serodiagnosis.[8] Difficulties in diagnosis may arise from the fact that the lesions in scabies closely resemble those from other papular dermatitis.[8] The diagnosis in this patient was achieved through clinical examination. Other laboratory tests (VDRL) were carried out on the patient to rule out sexually transmitted infections such as syphilis, which could also present with similar skin lesions.[9] It was also important to screen the patient for sexually transmitted disease because the possibility of sexual exposure was present being a young adolescent whose age group is prone to risky sexual behaviors.

Treatment using the correct drugs is important in all cases of scabies. As much as possible, treatment should also be given to all household contacts to prevent or contain transmission.[10] Treatment can be with topical or oral agents. Topical agents include Permethrin, Benzyl benzoate,

Crotamiton, and Gamma benzyl hexachloride. Oral drugs include Ivermectin. For this patient, Permethrin was used with good results. Oral Ivermectin was used in the mass treatment of the patient's neighbors with equally good outcomes.

Lessons learned/Recommendation:

Adequate treatment within the home, notification of cases, and contact tracing are useful measures to contain the spread of scabies in cases of mass infestation. Family physicians should pay closer attention to Neglected Tropical Diseases to reduce the disease burden.

References

1. Hay RJ, Steer AC, Engelman D, Walton S. Scabies in the developing world prevalence, complications and management. Clinical microbiology and infection. 2013; 18(4): 313 – 23

2. Karimhkani C, Colombara DV, Drucker AM, Norton SA, Hay R, Engelman D et al. The global burden of scabies: a cross-sectional analysis from the global burden of disease study 2015. The Lancet Infectious Diseases. 2017

3. GBD 2015 Disease and Injury Incidence and Prevalence Collaborators. Global, regional and national incidence, prevalence and years lived with disability for 310 diseases and injuries, 1990-2015: a systematic analysis for the global burden of disease study. The Lancet. 2015

4. Andrews RM, McCarthy J, Carapetis JR, Currie BJ. Skin disorders, including pyoderma, scabies, and tinea

infections. Pediatr Clin North Am. 2009; 56(6):1421-40.

5. Hegab DS, Kato AM, Kabbash IA, Dabish GM. Scabies among primary schoolchildren in Egypt: sociomedical environmental study in Kafr El-Sheikh administrative area. Clin Cosmet Investig Dermatol. 2015; 8:105–11.

6. Zayyid MM, Saadah RS, Adil AR, Rohela M, Jamaiah I. Prevalence of scabies and head lice among children in a welfare home in Pulau Pinang, Malaysia. Trop Biomed. 2010; 27: 442-446

7. Walton SF, Pizzuto S, Slender A, Viberg L, Holt D, Hales BJ, et al. Increased allergic immune response to *Sarcoptes scabiei* antigens in crusted versus ordinary scabies. Clin Vaccine Immunol. 2010; 17:1428-1438

8. Sambo MN, Idris SH, Umar AA, Olorukooba AA. Prevalence of scabies among school-aged children in

Katanga rural community in Kaduna state, Northwestern Nigeria. Ann Nigerian Med. 2012; 6:26-9

9. Ugbomoiko US, Oyedeji SA, Babamale OA, Heukelbach J. Scabies in resource-poor communities in Nasarawa state, Nigeria: epidemiology, clinical features and factors associated with infestation. Trop. Med. Infect. Dis. 2018. 3; 59

10. Kalu IE, Wagbatsoma V, Ogbaini-Emovon E, Nwadike VU, Ojide CK. Age and sex prevalence of infectious dermatoses among primary school children in a rural south-eastern Nigerian community. The Pan African Medical Journal. 2015; 20: 182

Chapter Fifteen

Acute Tonsillopharyngitis In A 10-Year-Old Boy

A 10-year-old male patient was seen at the General Hospital with fever and headache of 4 days' duration and neck pain of a day's duration.

He was apparently well until 4 days prior to the presentation when he developed a headache, which was intermittent, located frontally, and throbbing in nature. It was not associated with photophobia or dizziness. It was relieved temporarily by Acetaminophen tablets and rest. It was aggravated by movement of the head, noise, and light. Fever was gradual in onset, high-grade, continuous, and only temporarily relieved by Acetaminophen tablets. There was no aggravating factor. He did not have a history of cough, catarrh, chest pain, shortness of breath, ear pain ,discharge or dysuria. There was loss of appetite and vomiting. He had 4 episodes of vomiting and vomitus containing ingested meals and medication. There was no hemoptysis, diarrhea, blood in stool, or abdominal pain. A day before the presentation, he complained of pain in the throat and was unable to turn his neck from side to side. There was no difficulty in swallowing or, trauma to the neck, or history of travel. There was no history of body pain, difficulty in breathing, or dark urine.

His mother had given him Amartem tablets, P-alaxin tablets, Ciprotab tablets, Flagyl tablets, Loxagyl tablets, and Multivitamin syrup purchased at a patent drug store. She also gave him herbal medications, which were 'Agbo', pawpaw leaves, and Moringa tea. However, as his condition continued to deteriorate, a neighbor told her that the child's neck stiffness was due to meningitis, which would soon kill him. This prompted their presentation at the hospital. His mother was afraid that her son was dying because his symptoms were not improving despite all her interventions. Due to the illness, he missed school for some days. She felt that he was having a spiritual attack, manifesting as sickness, from her rivals in business. She expected him to be treated with drips.

His past medical and surgical history indicated that the patient had been admitted for acute tonsillitis some years prior to this visit. There was no history of surgeries or blood transfusions.

His birth was planned, and the pregnancy was uneventful, with his mother duly attending her scheduled antenatal visits. Delivery was at term, and his birth weight was 3.5kg. His developmental milestones were appropriate for his age. His immunization history showed he had completed immunization for his age, according to the National Program on Immunization. This was evident on his card.

The patient was a Primary Five pupil in a public primary school. He was the second of three children; he had a sister, and a brother aged 11 years and 7 years respectively. His father worked for the local government council as a revenue collector, while his mother was a trader in used clothes. Their source of healthcare financing was out of pocket. The family lived in a rented 2-bedroom apartment. Their source of drinking water was from a borehole, they used a water closet system for sewage disposal, and they had mosquito nets on the windows of their house. Using Evelyn Duvall's model, the family was at the school age children stage (stage 4).

The general physical examination showed the patient was acutely ill-looking and in pain, constantly holding his head and crying excessively. He was febrile with a temperature of 39.2°C. His anterior cervical lymph nodes were enlarged. There was no pallor, jaundice, dehydration, or pedal oedema. His weight was 39kg, which was normal for his age. He was fully conscious and alert. Kernig's and Brudzinski's signs were negative. The pupils were equal and reactive to light. Muscle tone, power, and reflexes were normal.

Examination of the eyes showed there were no swellings or discharge. His pupils reacted normally to light; the cup-disc ratio was within normal limits. Examination of the throat showed bilaterally inflamed and enlarged tonsils with purulent exudate covering the surface of both tonsils. The back of his throat was erythematous. His pulse rate was 100 beats per minute, with a regular rhythm and moderate volume. His blood pressure was 100/60 mmHg. The first and second heart sounds were heard on auscultation and there were no murmurs. His respiratory rate was 32 cycles per minute, there were resonant percussion notes, and his chest was clinically clear. Other systems were essentially normal.

A diagnosis of Acute Tonsillopharyngitis was made. The differential diagnosis was Cerebrospinal Meningitis.

Management:

The patient was admitted into the Children's ward, and the likely diagnoses and management plan were explained to the parents. Laboratory investigations done were complete blood count, cerebrospinal fluid (CSF) microscopy and culture, throat swab microscopy and culture, urinalysis, and blood film for malaria parasite. Lumbar puncture was done under aseptic conditions and yielded 1 ml of clear cerebrospinal fluid (CSF), which was not under pressure. It was sent to the laboratory for analysis. The investigation results showed there were no malaria parasites. Hematocrit level was 36%, and white cell count was $10.6 \times 10^9/l$ with a differential count of 67% neutrophils, 1% eosinophils, and 32% lymphocytes. The erythrocyte sedimentation rate was 10mm/hour (Westergren method). Cerebrospinal fluid analysis showed a cell count of 2.8 x 10^6/l, glucose 2.5mmol/l, and total protein 0.1g/l. Urine analysis results were within normal limits. His parents did not do the throat swab m/c/s, citing financial difficulty.

He was given intravenous Crystalline Penicillin 0.15mu/kg/day (6mu) in 4 divided doses 6 hourly for 48 hours, intravenous fluid 4.3% dextrose in 0.18% saline 500ml 12 hourly for 24 hours, and intramuscular Acetaminophen 300mg eight hourly for 24 hours. Six hours later, his temperature was 38.1°C and headache severity had reduced such that he was sleeping calmly.

First day on admission:

The patient had one episode of vomiting. Headache and neck pain were reduced. His temperature was 37.8⁰ C. Other vital signs were within normal limits. His medications were continued. His mother was encouraged to give him fluids and semi-solid foods as much as he could tolerate.

2nd – 3rd day of admission:

There were no new complaints. He was sitting up in bed and accepting semi-solid foods without vomiting.

His temperature was 37.2 ^{0} C, and other vital signs had been normal for more than 24 hours. Intravenous antibiotics were discontinued, and Amoxicillin/Clavulanate tablets 375mg twice daily for 5 days and multivitamin syrup were prescribed for a week. His parents were counseled on proper nutrition and hygiene, good health seeking behavior, prompt presentation to the hospital when sickness occurred, avoidance of self-medication and herbal remedies, as well as a regular check-up. Following this, he was discharged home and given a one-week appointment.

One-week follow-up:

When seen a week later, there were no new complaints. His physical examination findings were normal. His parents were counseled again on the importance of responsible self-medication. Following this, he was discharged.

Summary:

This was a 10-year-old boy who presented with fever, headache and neck pain. His condition was aggravated by a delay in presentation due to wrongful self-medication by his mother. He was diagnosed with Acute Tonsillopharyngitis and showed prompt response to treatment with antibiotics. Treatment also included health education on self-medication.

Discussion:

Acute tonsillopharyngitis is an infection of the pharynx and/or tonsils.[1] Usually referred to as sore throat, it is caused by inflammation of the back of the throat. Acute tonsillopharyngitis is very common in primary care and of great significance because of its distressing symptoms, potential spread of the causative organism, life-threatening complications resulting from the primary infection, and public health implications.[2] It is a common pathology among children and adolescents aged 5 – 15 years.[3]

The index patient was a 10-year-old boy who presented with symptoms and signs of acute tonsillopharyngitis.

Clinical manifestations include throat pain, fever, headache, and gastrointestinal symptoms.[4] Viruses, mainly rhinovirus, coronavirus, and adenovirus, have been identified as the predominant cause of this infection; however, studies have shown that in 37% of cases in children older than five years, group A β-hemolytic Streptococcus has been identified in the aetiology.[2] The clinical presentations of streptococcal and viral pharyngitis have considerably similar features; however, the onset of viral pharyngitis may be more gradual with symptomatology including cough, rhinorrhea and hoarseness.[4] In acute pharyngitis of streptococcal etiology, the presence of a purulent exudate usually reveals the diagnosis. This patient presented with fever, headache, and neck pain with signs of cervical lymph node enlargement. An examination of his throat also showed inflamed tonsils, which were covered by a purulent exudate, thus giving a pointer to his diagnosis.

Due to the high mortality rate, it was important to exclude cerebrospinal meningitis, which has similar symptoms,[5,] and so cerebrospinal fluid analysis was done in the index patient. Malaria also could present with similar features or as a comorbid condition with pharyngitis; however, the patient tested negative for malaria.[2,3]

The diagnosis can be done by throat culture or rapid diagnostic test.[6,7] Due to the disease being mainly of viral etiology, there have been many disputes regarding diagnostic microbiological tests as well as treatment with antibiotics.[7,8] In this patient, a throat culture, which could have been ideal was not done because his parents could not afford it; however based on his signs and symptoms and a high index of suspicion, a plausible diagnosis was made. The treatment of acute bacterial pharyngitis is done with antimicrobial therapy and usually produces good outcomes.[1,2] This was evident in this patient even though his treatment had been delayed because his mother went ahead to self-medicate.

Self-medication is the selection and use of non-prescription medicines by an individual's own initiatives to treat self-recognized illnesses or symptoms.[9] It is a common practice worldwide but more in resource-poor settings where it provides a lower-cost alternative for people of low socio-economic status. It can be appropriately used, however, and where this is done, it could lighten the demand for doctors and increase health awareness. However, it should be done responsibly with regard to indication, correct dosage and duration of illness.[9,10] This was not the case in this patient because prior to visiting the hospital, he had been exposed to an array of medicines, which caused an unnecessary delay in seeking proper medical care and a worsening of his clinical state. Wrongful self-medication can result in complications and even death in an individual.[9] Though the patient did not have complications, it was important to point this out to his mother to prevent future occurrences.

Lessons learned/Recommendation:

Wrong self-medication might just be the cause of many preventable deaths. It is recommended that at the clinics, family physicians should advocate for the avoidance of irresponsible self-medication by parents, particularly in the pediatric age group.

References

1. Regoli M, Chiappini E, Bonsignori F, Galli L, de Martino M. Update on the management of acute pharyngitis in children. Ital J Pediatr. 2011; 37:10.

2. Somro A. Akram M, Ibrahim-khan M, Asif HM, Sami A, Ali Shah SM et al. Pharyngitis and sore throat: A review. Africa Journal of Biotechnology. 2011; 10:33. 6190 -6197

3. Wu S, Peng X, Yang Z, et al. Estimated burden of group a streptococcal pharyngitis among children in Beijing, China. BMC Infect Dis. 2016; 16(1):452.

4. Shaikh N, Leonard E, Martin JM. Prevalence of Streptococcal Pharyngitis and Streptococcal Carriage in children: a meta-analysis. Pediatrics. 2010; 126: 4

5. Uzodimma CC, Dedeke FI, Nwadike V, Owolabi O, Arifalo G, Oduwole O. A study of group A streptococcal pharyngitis among 3–15-year-old children

attending clinics for an acute sore throat. Nig J Cardiol. 2017;14: 97-102

6. Weber R. Pharyngitis. Primary Care - Clinics in Office Practice. 2014; 41 (1), pp. 91-98.

7. Sadoh WE, Sadoh AE. Need for a clinical decisión rule for the management of pharyngitis in Nigeria. Nigerian Journal of Paediatrics. 2013; 40(1)

8. Ogah O, Adegbite G, Udoh S, Ogbodo E, Ogah F, Adesomowo A, *et al.* Chronic rheumatic heart disease in Abeokuta, Nigeria: Data from Abeokuta Heart Disease Registry. Niger J Cardiol 2014; 11:98-103.

9. Alano GM, Galafassil LM, Galato D, Trauthman SC. Responsible self-medication: review of the process of pharmaceutical attendance. BJPS. 2009; 45(4):626-633.

10. Kayalvizhi S, Senapathi R. Evaluation of the perception, attitude and practice of self-medication among business students in three selected cities in south

India. International Journal of Enterprise and Innovation Management Studies 2010; 1(3):40-44.

Chapter Sixteen

Cervical Spondylosis In A 70-Year-Old Woman

A 70-year-old female patient presented with recurrent neck pain of 1 year, headache of 1 week, and neck stiffness of 4 days. She was apparently well until the 1-year preceding presentation when she developed pain in the posterior area of her neck. This pain usually occurred intermittently; however, the present episode started 3 weeks prior to her visit. The onset was insidious, gradually increasing in intensity. The pain was sharp, continuous, radiated to the base of her head and shoulders, aggravated by movement of her neck and relieved initially by Paracetamol, application of a local pain-relieving ointment called 'Aboniki' and application of a hot water bottle at night when she went to bed. However, there was eventually no relief. About 4 days before the presentation, she developed neck stiffness and was unable to turn her neck from side to side. There was associated numbness of her fingertips, which occurred intermittently. There was a history of similar complaints which occurred about a year prior to this presentation. There was no history of trauma, falls, fever, vomiting, swellings on the head and neck, or travel to meningitis-endemic regions. There were also no arm or leg pains and no urinary symptoms. There was no history of cough, chest pain, difficulty in breathing, palpitations, abdominal pain or swelling, constipation, diarrhea, yellowness of the eyes, breast pain, breast masses, vaginal bleeding, or joint swelling. The patient felt that her symptoms were due to a bad sleep posture. Her fear was that the numbness in her fingers indicated a very serious problem, and this was her immediate reason for presentation. The illness had made her unable to attend her church activities, which were a source of joy for her. She expected that she would be treated adequately with due consideration of her financial state. She had delayed presenting to the hospital because she was apprehensive about treatment costs.

Her past medical and surgical history showed she was a hypertensive patient who was diagnosed about twenty years earlier and was taking antihypertensive drugs – Amlodipine and Moduretic. She had good control. She had undergone three Caesarean section operations. The patient was a Para 3^{+0} woman with all children alive. She had been post-menopausal for about twenty-two years. She had never done a Pap smear.

She was the sixth of eight children, three males and five females. Both parents were deceased. She also had four deceased older siblings, all of whom had died of natural causes. She had three children, two males and one female, and six grandchildren. She was a widow who had been married to a lawyer for forty-five years, and he had died five years earlier of natural causes. She was a retired civil servant whose source of income was mainly from her pension. She lived in a one-storey building with her housekeeper. The patient was a non-smoker and had never taken any tobacco products in her life. She did not take alcohol. Her source of healthcare financing was out-of-pocket. Her family APGAR assessment was eight out of ten, indicating a highly functional family. Her family stage, according to Evelyn Duvall's family staging, was 8 (ageing family).

A physical examination revealed an elderly woman in pain. She was afebrile and not pale. There was no icterus, cyanosis, peripheral lymphadenopathy, or pedal oedema. There was no evidence of muscle wasting on the neck. There were no scars, scarification marks, swellings or sinuses. Tenderness was elicited on the lateral parts of the neck. There was a limited range of movement due to pain.

She had reduced sensation on the C6 and C7 dermatomes of the upper limbs.

She was conscious, alert, and well-oriented. There was no sign of meningeal irritation or cranial nerve abnormality. Her pulse rate was 84 beats per minute with a regular rhythm and full volume. The blood pressure was 140/80 mmHg. Her jugular venous pressure was not raised. Her apex beat was at the fifth left intercostal space on the mid-clavicular line. The first and second heart sounds were only heard. The abdomen examination showed her abdomen was full, soft and moved with respiration. There was no area of tenderness and no organomegaly. Her bowel sounds were normoactive. Examination of other systems revealed normal findings.

A diagnosis of Cervical Spondylosis was made.

Management:

The findings, diagnosis, and management plan were explained to the patient. She appealed that all drugs and tests should be prescribed with due consideration of the costs, as she relied on her pension and was not willing to overburden her children financially. She was given a stat dose of Diclofenac 75 mg intramuscularly and tablets of Acetaminophen 1000mg orally for immediate relief of pain. A plain X-ray of the cervical spine (anterior-posterior and lateral views) was done. The cervical spine x-ray showed osteophyte growth at the anterior and posterior parts of C5, C6, and C7 vertebral bodies and reduction of the C5/C6 and C6/C7 intervertebral disc spaces.

The drugs prescribed for her were tablets Arthrotec 75 (Diclofenac 75mg/Misoprostol 200µg) 12-hourly orally for 5 days and tablets Tizanidine hydrochloride (Sirdalud) 4mg twice daily orally for 7 days. A soft neck collar was to be applied for 6 weeks. She was advised to eat sufficiently before drug ingestion and report immediately to the hospital if she had gastrointestinal symptoms like upper abdominal pain, heartburn or vomiting. She was also advised to swallow the Arthrotec tablet whole and not crush, chew, or break the pill. Subsequently, she was given a one-week appointment.

One-week follow-up visit:

She was seen a week later. She reported that neck pain had reduced moderately. She had not been consistent with applying the neck collar because it was uncomfortable, and she was self-conscious about wearing it in public. She was gently advised to apply the neck collar consistently as it would help in reducing neck stiffness. There were no complaints of gastrointestinal symptoms. She was told to continue her medications for another week and given a one-week clinic appointment. The patient was requested to attend the clinic with her daughter and housekeeper.

Two weeks follow-up visit:

She made her scheduled visit in the company of her daughter and housekeeper. She complained of occasional numbness in her extremities. There was no neck pain. Her daughter was encouraged to support her financially. The patient's daughter revealed that a major challenge they had with her mother was her refusal to accept financial support from her children. The patient was counseled to allow her children to support her financially and relieve her of undue psychological stress. Her daughter insisted that she would bear the cost of her treatment. Her housekeeper was also encouraged to assist her with activities of daily living, ensure that she adhered to her medications, and prevent her from lifting heavy loads. She was given tablets Neurovite forte once daily for 4 weeks and to discontinue Arthrotec and Sirdalud. In addition, she was to continue applying her neck collar. Subsequently, she was given a one-month appointment.

Six-weeks follow-up visit:

The patient was seen a month after her last visit in the company of her daughter. There were no complaints of neck pain, stiffness, or numbness of her fingers. She admitted that she had stopped using her neck collar a week earlier. She was advised on good nutrition and regular medical check-ups at the geriatric clinic. She was taking her antihypertensive medications regularly. The patient was happy that her treatment had been affordable and not burdened her financially. Following this, she was discharged.

Summary:

A 70-year-old woman presented with complaints of neck pain and stiffness. She desired to have good clinical care but was concerned about the cost of the treatment being a retiree. She was given medical and conservative management.

Discussion:

Cervical spondylosis is a chronic degenerative condition of the cervical spine that affects the vertebral bodies and intervertebral discs of the neck, leading to herniated intervertebral disks, osteophytes, and ligament hypertrophy. Compression of the nerve roots and spinal cord may result from this process.[1] The global incidence of cervical spondylosis has been reported at 13.1%.[2,3,4] In Nigeria, a study done in the south western region reported a prevalence of 10.7%.[5] It is the most frequent cause of spinal cord dysfunction in patients older than 55 years.[6] The index patient was a 70-year old woman and was within the age range for this condition.

Cervical spondylosis can be caused by different factors. These include injury to the cervical spine from falls and road traffic accidents and lifting heavy loads. Risk factors include age, genetic factors such as family history of cervical spondylosis, smoking, unhealthy working position, menopause, obesity, and overweight.[7,8] Age has been found to be the main risk factor as the risk increases with ageing.[4] In this patient, the risk factors were age and menopause. Her health education also included counseling on the dangers of lifting heavy loads.

The clinical presentation may take various patterns, which could range from asymptomatic to very severe. The symptoms include neck pain, which is the most common symptom, neck stiffness, numbness or tingling at the shoulders or arms, muscle weakness, and headaches. Symptoms that may occur less frequently are loss of balance, and loss of bowel control. In this patient, neck pain was the major complaint with associated occasional numbness of her fingers.

Diagnosis of this condition can be achieved using X-rays, computed tomography scans, magnetic resonance imaging, and myelography. Nerve function tests can also be done, and these include electromyography and nerve conduction studies. In the management of this patient, an x-ray of the cervical spine was utilized to aid her diagnosis. This was the most cost-effective option for her and was considered because she had been concerned about the cost involved in the management of her disease.

Treatment can be achieved with medications, surgery, or physiotherapy. A common non-operative treatment for cervical spondylosis is neck immobilization with a neck collar. Medications include non-steroidal anti-inflammatory drugs, corticosteroids, muscle relaxants, anti-seizure drugs, and anti-depressants. The patient was treated with non-steroidal anti-inflammatory drugs and muscle relaxants (tizanidine hydrochloride) while a neck collar was applied for six weeks. Some patients also use home treatments in the management of their symptoms. These include hot balms, warm compresses, ice packs and massage. This patient had applied a hot balm (Aboniki) for many weeks to relieve her neck pain.

The challenges in the management of this patient, who was of the geriatric age group, included inaccurate perceptions of her symptoms and treatment, difficulty in compliance with medications, and socio-economic disadvantage. She was a retiree who depended on a moderate government stipend for sustenance and refused to accept financial support from her children because she felt it would be burdensome on them. As such, all treatment modalities used were affordable with optimal efficacy. Polypharmacy was avoided as much as possible because of the possibility of adverse drug reactions common in this age group.

Lessons Learned/Recommendations:

Chronic pain, such as seen in cervical spondylosis, can be a source of great financial distress to geriatric patients. Thus, it is important for family physicians to advocate for healthcare insurance for the elderly to mitigate catastrophic health expenses.

References

1. Xiong W, Li F, Guan H. Tetraplegia after thyroidectomy in a patient with cervical spondylosis: a case report and literature review. Medicine (Baltimore) 2015;94: e524

2. Schairer WW, Carrer A, Lu M, Hu SS. The increased prevalence of cervical spondylosis in patients with adult thoracolumbar spinal deformity. J Spinal Disord Tech. 2014;27: E305–E308

3. Global, regional, and national incidence, prevalence, and years lived with disability for 301 acute and chronic diseases and injuries in 188 countries, 1990–2013: a systematic analysis for the Global Burden of Disease Study 2013. Lancet. 2015; 386:743–800.

4. Yang W, Lu J, Weng J, Jia W, Ji L, Xiao J, et al. Prevalence of diabetes among men and women in China. N Engl J Med. 2010; 362:1090–1101.

5. Oguntona SA. Cervical spondylosis in southwest Nigerian farmers and female traders. Ann Afr Med. 2014; 13:61–64

6. Goode AP, Freburger J, Carey T. Prevalence, practice patterns, and evidence for chronic neck pain. Arthritis Care Res (Hoboken) 2010; 62:1594–1601

7. Singh S, Kumar D, Kumar S. Risk factors in cervical spondylosis. J Clin Orthop Trauma. 2014; 5:221–226.

8. Iheukwumere N, Okoye E. Prevalence of symptomatic cervical spondylosis in a Nigerian tertiary health institution. Trop J Med Res. 2014; 17:25-7

9. Breivik H, Eisenberg E, O'Brien T. The individual and societal burden of chronic pain in Europe: the case for strategic prioritization and action to improve knowledge and availability of appropriate care. *BMC Public Health.* 2013; 13:1229

10. Igwe AA, Okoye GC, Eyichukwu GO, Ezema CI, Egwuonwu AV, Onwujekwe O. Treatment of cervical

spondylosis in southeast Nigeria. BJMMR. 2016;16(7): 1-7.

Chapter Seventeen

Depression Following Burns Injury In A Welder

A 43-year-old male patient was brought to the clinic with complaints of loss of interest in activities, inability to sleep, and weight loss of three months' duration.

He was apparently well until three months prior to the presentation when his wife noticed that the patient had withdrawn socially and was not interested in activities that would ordinarily interest him. On many days, he would not go to work, calling in sick when he was not sick, and would lock himself indoors without going out or eating. He was an avid soccer fan who would never miss a soccer match at his favorite soccer club but now showed no interest in soccer. He refused to attend his local club meetings even though he was the club chairman and would not pick up calls from his friends. There was difficulty in initiating and maintaining sleep. He usually had about 3 hours of sleep at night, waking up at about 4 a.m. in the morning, unable to sleep anymore. As a result, he was not refreshed in the mornings and was always fatigued.

There was loss of appetite and weight loss which was evident in his clothes that were now very loose-fitting. His colleagues and friends had remarked on his weight loss. There was no history of cough, fever, excessive night sweats, lumps in any part of his body, abdominal swelling, yellowness of the eyes, or palpitations. He was constantly restless and usually told his wife that he felt worthless and unfulfilled in life. There was no loss of memory, no suicidal ideation, no history of psychoactive substance use, and no history of visual or auditory hallucinations.

He stated that he was unhappy because of a fire incident he was involved in about seven months earlier. A large container of thinner had exploded close to him as he tried to weld pieces of metal. He sustained burns on his thighs, which had healed with unsightly scars. His company had refused to pay him any compensation for this issue, and he felt unfairly treated. The patient feared that he would lose his job because he felt the company placed no value on his life. His idea was that his issues with the company were due to a spiritual attack. The illness had greatly inhibited his social life. He expected to be given medications that would make him sleep well at night and make him happy.

His past medical and surgical history showed there was no history of hypertension, diabetes, asthma, sickle cell, epilepsy, or mental illness. There was no history of surgeries. He was not on any drugs of chronic use and had no allergies.

He was the first child in a family of four children, one male and three females. His parents were alive and well. He was a welder at a generator assembly plant and was married to a

35-year-old foodstuff trader. They had three children, one male and two female, all of whom were primary school pupils. They lived in their own home, which was a 3-bedroom apartment within his family compound. He occasionally indulged in alcoholic drinks like beer and local gin. The patient did not smoke or take illicit substances. Assessment of family Apgar showed a score of 8 which was indicative of a highly functional family. He had a cordial relationship with his extended family members and colleagues at work.

He was the chairman of a local cooperative society and had a good relationship with his fellow members. He had no history of violence or altercations with law enforcement agents and was generally regarded as a friendly and law-abiding person. A physical examination showed a healthy young man who was afebrile and not pale. He was not icteric or cyanosed. His weight was 75kg. There was no peripheral lymphadenopathy and no pedal oedema.

The mental state examination showed the patient was well-dressed, wearing a clean shirt over denim trousers. However, he was not well-kempt as he had not shaved and did not cut his hair. He was calm but avoided eye contact and was not forthcoming during the examination. He described his mood as low. His affect was appropriate and in congruence with his mood. His speech had a low volume but was coherent and at a normal rate. The stream, form, and possession of his thoughts were normal. There was no abnormal perception. He was attentive to each question with equal concentration. His immediate recall short term and long-term memory were normal. His judgment also was normal, and he had an insight into his problem.

His pulse rate was 70 beats per minute with a full volume and regular rhythm. There was synchrony of the peripheral pulses. The patient's blood pressure was 120/70 mmHg. The first and second heart sounds were only heard. The respiratory rate was 20 cycles per minute. There was equal chest expansion, percussion notes were resonant, and breath sounds were vesicular.

His abdomen was flat, soft, and moved with respiration. There were no areas of tenderness, and there were no palpably enlarged organs. His bowel sounds were normoactive. There were large, raised scars on the inner parts of both thighs. There was no tenderness elicited on the limbs. He had complete range of motion on all joints. Motor and sensory examinations were normal.

A diagnosis of Major Depression was made based on Diagnostic and Statistical Manual V criteria for depression.

Management:

The patient's diagnosis and management plan were explained to him and his wife. He was informed that his management would be both pharmacological and non-pharmacological. He was told that his health issues were likely precipitated by the fire incident and subsequent work-related issues. He was told that setbacks were bound to happen in life, but a positive response was needed to overcome them. As such, withdrawal from social activities, family, and friends was not a good approach to adopt when confronted with problems. He was encouraged to resume his social activities and advised on healthy eating, exercise, and sleep hygiene.

Subsequently, medications were prescribed, which included bromazepam tablets 3mg orally at night for 5 days, sertraline tablets 25mg daily orally for six weeks, and multivitamins tablets one twice orally for two weeks. He was informed about the side effects of sertraline, being nausea, drowsiness, diarrhea, and skin rash, and was advised to take the medication at night. The patient was co-managed with the clinical psychologist, who administered psychotherapy in the form of cognitive behavioral therapy on him. It involved helping him focus on replacing his negative feelings of guilt with positive thoughts. He was encouraged to focus on his achievements in life, family, career and social circle. He was given a one-week clinic appointment, and a medical report was issued to him.

One week follow-up visit:

He attended the clinic in the company of his wife. He still complained of early morning awakening but stated that he felt refreshed when he woke up. He also complained of loose stools; however, stool frequency had not increased. Bromazepam tablets 3mg daily orally were prescribed for 5 days. He was encouraged to continue his medication. The patient was scheduled for another follow-up visit in one month.

One-month follow-up visit:

Here, the patient reported a better sleep pattern and better appetite. His weight was 78kg. He reported that he had engaged in fruitful negotiations with his employers, who agreed to pay him some compensation for the workplace accident. He was eager to resume work. He was asked to complete his medications and return in 3 months. He was also encouraged to resume work if he was in a good mental state.

Three months follow-up visit:

At this visit, the patient had no complaints. He described his mood as happy, and his affect showed the same. He was counseled to observe safety regulations at work to avoid occupational hazards, and maintain healthy lifestyle practices in diet, exercise, and sleep hygiene. Subsequently, he was discharged.

Summary:

A 43-year company welder presented with a loss of interest in activities, inability to sleep, and weight loss. His mental illness was possibly triggered by a fire incident in the workplace in which he was involved. He was treated with drugs and psychotherapy.

Discussion:

Depression is defined as a mood disorder that has affective, cognitive as well as physical signs and symptoms.[1] It is the leading cause of mental health-related disease burden globally, affecting an estimated 322 million people.[2] In Nigeria, a population-based survey reported 3.1% and 1.1% lifetime and 12-month prevalence of depression.[3]

Depression can be classified as major depression or minor depression.[1,4,5] This is usually determined by a collection of symptoms.

According to the Diagnostic and Statistical Manual of Mental Disorders, 5th edition, text revision (DSM-V-TR), the criteria for major depression includes persistently depressed mood, diminished ability to take pleasure in activities, feelings of worthlessness and guilt, poor concentration, suicidal ideation, excessive tiredness, significantly altered appetite and weight, sleep alterations, and psychomotor agitation or retardation.[1] A person is judged as having major depression in the presence of at least five of these criteria daily for two weeks or longer and should not be the direct result of a drug or medical condition.[1,4] The index patient presented with most of these criteria, thereby necessitating the diagnosis of major depressive disorder.

A burn injury is a traumatic event with effects that can profoundly affect the physical and psychological aspects of the injured person's life. A traumatic event, as defined by the Diagnostic and Statistical Manual for Psychiatry 5th Edition (DSM V), is an event in which a person witnessed that involved actual or threatened death or serious injury to self or others and that the event was responded to with intense fear, helplessness, or horror.[1,] Psychological effects may include depression, mood disorders, and anxiety disorders [7, 8] The onset of this patient's illness was triggered by an explosion causing burns which eventually resulted in depression. These reactions highlighted the connection between burns and depression.

The diagnosis of major depression is based on a patient's self-reported experiences, behavior reported by friends or relatives, and mental state examination.

In this patient, his spouse presented a detailed account of the patient's illness experience, which aided in the diagnosis and management. Treatment of depression can be achieved using several antidepressant medications, psychotherapy and counseling.[10]

Medications include selective serotonin reuptake inhibitors (SSRI), tricyclic antidepressants, monoamine oxidase inhibitors, and selective serotonin-norepinephrine reuptake inhibitors.[10] Sertraline, a SSRI, was used for the patient because of its relatively mild side effects and its reduced toxicity in a case of overdose. The types of psychotherapy include cognitive behavioral therapy (CBT), interpersonal psychotherapy, and problem-solving therapy.[10] CBT was used in this patient's treatment because it is considered the most evidence-based psychological therapy for depression.[10]

Lessons Learned/Recommendations:

Most patients who present with depression at the family medicine clinic may go undiagnosed. Thus, family physicians should be attentive to psychological symptoms as much as to physical symptoms in order not to miss the diagnosis. There is a need for government to ensure the availability of good mental health services.

References

1. The American Psychiatric Association. Depressive disorders. Diagnostic and Statistical Manual of Mental Disorders. Psychiatric News: American Psychiatric Association (DSM Library); 2013. Available from https://www.doi.org/10.1176

2. Ferrari AJ, Charlson FJ, Norman RE, Patten SB, Freedman G, Murray CJ, et al. Burden of depressive disorders by country, sex, age and year: findings from the global burden of disease study 2010. PLoS Med. 2013;10: e1001547

3. Gureje O, Uwakwe R, Oladeji B, Makanjuola VO, Esan O, Moormal H, et al. Depression in adult Nigerians: results from the Nigerian survey of mental health and well-being. J Affect Disord. 2010; 120:158-64

4. Sarokhani D, Delpisheh A, Veisani Y, Sarokhani M, Esmaeli M, Sayehmiri K. Prevalence of depression among university students: A systematic review and

meta-analysis study. Depression *Research and Treatment.* 2013.

5. Asibong UE, Udonwa NE, Okokon IB, Gyuse AN, Aluka T, Ekpe EE. Patient characteristics that may predict the likelihood of the presence of mental health problems in patients attending general outpatient clinic in a tertiary hospital in South-South Nigeria. *Ment Health Fam Med* 2010 Sep;7(3):169-177

6. Goar SG, Obembe A, Audu MD, Agbir MT. Utilization of health care services by depressed patients attending the general out-patients department of the Jos University Teaching Hospital, Jos, Nigeria. Niger J Clin Pract. 2012; 15:59-62.

7. Oladele AO, Olabanji JK. Burns in Nigeria: a review. *Ann Burns Fire Disasters.* 2010; 23(3):120-7.

8. Egwuonwu CC, Kanma-Okafor OJ, Ogunyemi AO, Yusuf HO, Adeyemi JD. Depression-related knowledge, attitude, and help-seeking behavior among

residents of Surulere Local Government Area, Lagos State, Nigeria. J Clin Sci. 2019; 16:49-56.

9. Ademola AD, Boima V, Odusola AO, Agyekun F, Nwafor CE, Salako BL. Prevalence and determinants of depression among patients with hypertension: a cross-sectional comparison study in Ghana and Nigeria. Niger J Clin Pract. 2019; 22:558-65

10. Ng CW, How CH, Ng YP. Managing depression in primary care. Singapore Med J. 2017;58(8):459-466.

Chapter Eighteen

Post-Traumatic Stress Disorder Following Intimate Partner Violence In A Female Civil Servant

A 32-year-old female patient presented to the clinic with recurrent nightmares, persistent fear, and difficulty in concentration for 2 months.

She was apparently well until two months before the presentation when she started having recurrent nightmares where she would see her estranged husband chasing her with knives and, in some cases, killing her. These nightmares initially occurred about two nights per week but increased in frequency and intensity to almost every night. She usually woke up with feelings of dread, terror and generalized weakness.

She also complained of flashbacks of the domestic violence episodes she experienced in her marriage to her former husband. Due to these flashbacks, she had developed fear which was persistent at all times of the day and night thus, she avoided driving on former familiar routes and going to places where she used to go with her former husband, such as church, their children's school and office (as they both worked in the same place). Her colleague reported that she had difficulty concentrating on her job, was always sad, withdrawn, and easily startled by trivial sounds such as people laughing. She also missed work regularly, and this had become a source of concern to her colleagues which prompted them to encourage her to seek expert medical care. She had divorced her husband two months earlier due to issues of domestic violence. He had repeatedly hit her, bitten her with his teeth, poured hot soup on her, and even tried to strangle her to death on three occasions. At the last incidence of domestic violence, which preceded her divorce, he beat her until she lost consciousness and suffered a miscarriage. She had a previous history of rape by a senior student in secondary school when she was 14 years old. She was afraid that her husband would eventually kill her and her two children as he was constantly sending her threatening messages. She blamed herself for marrying him without investigating his background carefully, and she expected to be given drugs that would treat the nightmares and help her forget her traumatic ordeal.

She complained of fever, loss of appetite, and bitterness of the mouth. There was no cough, chest pain, difficulty in breathing, abdominal pain, or urinary symptoms. There was no weight loss, polydipsia, or polyphagia.

In her past medical and surgical history, she had been admitted several times for injuries due to domestic violence, which included lacerations, ankle sprain, and blunt trauma. She had no history of hypertension, diabetes, asthma, epilepsy or sickle cell disease. She had no history of psychiatric illness or suicide attempts. She was a Para 3^{+1} (2 alive) woman. Her children had been born through spontaneous vaginal delivery. She had suffered a miscarriage at 12 weeks gestation, about five months prior to her visit, following a violent beating by her husband. She was having her menstrual period at the time of her presentation. Her menstrual flow lasted for 5 days, and her menstrual cycle was 30 days.

There was no history of dysmenorrhea. She was not on any form of contraception. She was the third child in a family of five children. Her mother was alive, but her father was deceased following injuries from a road traffic accident. She was an accountant at a tertiary hospital and had been married for six years before getting divorced. She lived with her children in a rented two-bedroom home. She had a good relationship with all her siblings but was closest to her immediate elder sister and mother.

Her sources of psychological support were her family and church. She was regarded by her colleagues as a decent, law-abiding woman. She did not take alcohol or tobacco in any form.

A physical examination showed a young woman who was mildly febrile with a body temperature of 37.8^0C. She was not pale, icteric, cyanosed, or dehydrated. There were numerous scars on her arms, legs, and back, showing evidence of physical assault. There were also bite marks on the right upper region of her back.

The mental state examination revealed she was dressed in casual mid-length trousers and a tee shirt. She was not well-kempt, as evidenced by her uncombed hair. Her speech was normal in rate and volume; she described her mood as 'alright', and her affect was mildly blunted. She was cooperative coherent, and the stream, form, and possession of her thoughts were normal. She denied auditory or visual hallucinations. She also denied suicidal or homicidal ideation. Her insight and judgment were normal. Her immediate recall and short term and long-term memory were also normal.

In the central nervous system examination, there was no evidence of meningeal irritation or cranial nerve deficit. Tone, power, and reflexes in all her limbs were normal. The sensation was normal. Her pulse rate was 98 beats per minute, regular and of full volume. Her blood pressure was 130/80 mmHg. Her apex beat was at the fifth left intercostal space, mid-clavicular line. Her first and second heart sounds were heard. Her respiratory rate was 20 cycles per minute. Her chest expansion was equal, and she had vesicular breath sounds. The gastrointestinal system examination showed her abdomen was flat, soft, and moved with respiration. There was slight tenderness in the epigastric region. No organ was palpable, and bowel sounds were normoactive.

A diagnosis of post-traumatic stress disorder due to intimate partner violence was made.

Management:

Her diagnosis and treatment plan were gently discussed with her. Treatment commenced with tablets Paroxetine 25 mg orally daily for one month and tablets Bromazepam 3mg orally for five nights. She was tested for malaria parasites, which was positive, and commenced on tablets of Artemether-Lumefantrine twice daily for three days.

Cognitive behavioral therapy was discussed with the patient, where she would be co-managed with the clinical psychologist. She was told that it was a treatment approach that would teach the patient how to cope with her illness through relaxation techniques as well as setting up anxiety-provoking scenes where she would be gradually exposed to similar ordeals like what she passed through (although in a controlled manner) until she became desensitized to the situation and was no longer afraid. She agreed to commence this treatment, noting that she hoped it would give her relief from the nightmares, which had become very distressing. She was given a one-week clinic appointment and issued a one- week sick leave.

1st follow-up visit:

She returned to the clinic after a week for her first follow-up visit, accompanied by her mother. She reported fatigue due to her medication but affirmed that her sleep had improved that week. She was advised to increase her fluid intake and rest more.

2nd follow-up visit:

She was seen two weeks later. She had commenced therapy with the clinical psychologist. She reported that there was no improvement in her condition, as she still had nightmares and flashbacks. Thus, she did not want to continue therapy. She also constantly received threatening messages from her husband, who threatened to physically confront her in the office and embarrass her. She had decided that she would resign from her job and relocate to another city where most of her siblings lived. However, she was encouraged not to resign as this would negatively impact her finances and economic well-being as her job was her only source of income.

Following this, the writer intervened by informing the hospital authorities, and the patient's former husband (who was also a staff) was issued a strict warning to refrain from assaulting or embarrassing her. He would face severe penalties if he failed to comply. During this visit, she was given reading materials on domestic violence and shown pictures of survivors of domestic violence.

On her subsequent clinic visits, which spanned over four months, she was advised to gradually begin to visit places that she had been avoiding. Over these sessions, the patient's condition gradually improved. She received her medication for three months. Her nightmares and flashbacks reduced considerably, and she reported feeling less startled by sudden loud sounds. She also admitted that she was no more burdened by the guilt of having dissolved her marriage and had decided to join an advocacy group to help other women who had undergone intimate partner violence. Regarding avoidance, although she was no longer afraid, she preferred to keep a distance from her former partner, given his violent nature. The patient's follow-up is still in progress.

Summary:

A 31-year-old accountant diagnosed with post-traumatic stress disorder following intimate partner violence. She was managed in conjunction with the clinical psychologist. Her therapy included drugs and cognitive behavioral therapy.

Discussion:

Posttraumatic stress disorder (PTSD) is a mental health condition that develops after a sudden and life-threatening event, involving high intensity fear of dying, helplessness, and loss of control.[1] It has been estimated that up to 10% of the population has been affected by the condition and treated; however, a greater proportion have gone unrecognized.[2] The patient was a young, recently divorced woman who had experienced severe physical assault, which was life-threatening, by her former husband.

PTSD can affect any person who has been involved in a significant or even non-significant traumatic event. However, not everyone who has experienced trauma will develop the condition. The predisposing factors may include family dysfunction, comorbid mental health disorders like depression, substance misuse, intense, long-lasting trauma, occupations that are exposed to trauma like military occupation, lack of good social support, and previous history of abuse.[3] The likely risk factor in the index patient was a previous history of sexual abuse, as she had been raped when she was a teenager. Causes include stressful experiences like combat exposure, accidents, fire, natural disasters, plane crashes, kidnapping, armed robbery, life-threatening medical diagnoses, childhood abuse, and intimate partner violence.[2,3] The index patient's condition was caused by intimate partner violence.

Intimate partner violence refers to any behavior within an intimate relationship that causes physical, psychological or sexual harm to those in the relationship.[4] These behaviors include physical violence, sexual abuse, emotional abuse, and controlling behaviours.[4] Intimate partner violence is widespread in all countries as estimates from a World Health Organization multi-country study show that 13-61% of women have experienced physical violence by a partner, 6-59% have experienced sexual violence, and 20-75% have had emotionally abusive acts.[4] Some factors that predispose a woman's increased likelihood of experiencing violence by her partner include low educational level, sexual abuse during childhood, exposure to other forms of prior violence, acceptance of violence, and economic stress.[5,6] In this patient's case, she had been exposed to sexual abuse as a young girl and also had shown acceptance of her husband's violence during her marriage in order to keep her family together.

According to the Diagnostic and Statistical Manual of Mental Disorders-5 (DSM-5), the diagnosis of PTSD requires certain criteria, which include exposure to a traumatic event, re-experience of the event in the form of nightmares or flashbacks, avoidance of event-related stimuli, persistence of negative feelings and thoughts about oneself that began or worsened after the event, and trauma-related arousal or hyperactivity.[7] The symptoms should have been present for at least one month and should interfere with the patient's daily functioning. The patient had most of these symptoms, and they had been present for two months, thus confirming the diagnosis. Treatment of PTSD is usually done using a variety of methods.

Treatment methods include medications and psychotherapy, a combination of both being the most effective method. Medications include antidepressants, anxiolytics, and antipsychotics, and psychotherapy could be cognitive behavioral therapy, family therapy, counseling, and debriefing. The patient was treated using medications and psychotherapy. She had a good treatment outcome.

Lessons Learnt/Recommendations:

Post-traumatic stress disorder (PTSD) is more common in our environment than what appears. Victims of intimate partner violence who present to the clinic should be screened for PTSD.

References

1. Becker KD, Steuwig J, McCloskey LA. Traumatic stress symptoms of women exposed to different forms of childhood victimization and intimate partner violence. Journal of Interpersonal Violence. 2010;25(9)

2. Bell KM, Orcutt HK. Posttraumatic stress disorder and male perpetrated intimate partner violence. JAMA. 2009;302(5):562-564

3. Taft CT, Watkins LE, Stafford J, Street AE, & Monson CM. Posttraumatic stress disorder and intimate relationship problems: A meta-analysis. Journal of Consulting and Clinical Psychology. 2009;79(1):22-33.

4. Nwoga CN, Audu MD, Obembe A. Prevalence and correlates of posttraumatic stress disorder among medical students in the University of Jos, Nigeria. Niger J Clin Pract. 2016; 19: 595-9

5. Cronholm PF, Fogarty CT, Ambuel B, Harrison SL. Intimate partner violence. Am Fam Physician. 2011;83(10): 1165-1172

6. Balogun MO, Owoaje ET, Fawole OI. Intimate partner violence in South-western Nigeria: are there rural-urban differences? Women and Health. 2012;5297):627-645

7. American Psychiatric Association. Diagnostic and Statistical Manual of Mental Disorders, 5th Edn. Washington, DC.

8. Hetrick SE, Purcell R, Garner B, Parslow R. Combined pharmacotherapy and psychological therapies for post-traumatic stress disorder. Cochrane Database Syst Rev. 2010;7(7).

9. Tagurum YO, Chirdan OO, Obindo T, Bello DA, Afolaranmi OT, et al. Prevalence of violence and symptoms of post-traumatic stress disorder among victims of ethno-religious conflict in Jos. Nigeria. J Psychiatry 2015;18: 178.

10. Kar N. Cognitive behavioural therapy for the treatment of post-traumatic stress disorder: a review. Neuropsychiatr Dis Treat. 2011; 7:167–181.

11. Cohen JA, Mannarino AP, Iyengar S. Community treatment of posttraumatic stress disorder for children exposed to intimate partner violence: A randomized controlled trial. Arch Pediatr Adolesc Med. 2011; 165(1):16–21.

Chapter Nineteen

The Importance Of Adequate Counselling In The Family Planning Clinic

A 42-year-old female client visited the clinic to request for reversal of the contraceptive method.

The client had no medical problem but came to request for reversal of the contraceptive method she was using. She was newly married to her current spouse and desired to have children for him. She had been previously married but had lost her spouse to an unknown illness about eight years earlier. That marriage lasted twelve years and produced three children. After her last child was born, they decided not to have any more children and so she tied her tubes. Shortly after, her husband died.

About six years later, she met her current husband, and they got married. She desired to have children with him to consolidate their union. Her fear was that since he was ten years younger than her, the marriage would break up if they did not have children. She had the idea that all contraceptive methods were reversible, and her expectation was that surgery would be done to untie her tubes. There was no abnormal vaginal discharge, vaginal itching, breast pain or swelling,

Her past medical and surgical history revealed there was no history of hypertension, epilepsy, diabetes, asthma, or sickle cell disease. She had undergone two Caesarean deliveries with no complications. She frequently ingested vitamin supplements. There was no history of allergies to any drugs.

Her obstetric and gynecological history revealed she was P_3^{+0} (all alive). Her menarche occurred at 13 years of age. Her menstrual flow lasted between 3-4 days and her cycle length was 25-27 days. She had done bilateral tubal ligation at a hospital in Sierra Leone about eight years earlier. At that time, she had not planned to have more children and was also relocating to Sweden. There was no history of dysmenorrhea or menorrhagia. She had her last Pap smear a year earlier.

In her family and social history, she was from a large polygamous home. Her father had eight wives and over forty children. She could not ascertain her position in that family. Her own mother, however, had nine children (3 boys and six girls), and she was the fifth child. She worked as a caregiver for people with disabilities in Sweden. From her first marriage, she had three daughters aged 20, 19, and 17 years. She was currently married to a 32-year-old pastor who was based in Calabar. They had met when he accompanied the senior pastor of his church to Sweden on ministry work. He intended to relocate to Sweden to be with her. She took alcohol occasionally and did not take tobacco in any form.

In the review of systems, there was no fever, headache, cough, chest pain, difficulty in breathing, abdominal pain, swellings on any part of the body, or urinary symptoms.

The physical examination revealed a healthy-looking woman who was in no obvious distress. She was afebrile and was not pale, icteric, dehydrated, or cyanosed. There was no significant peripheral lymphadenopathy or pedal oedema. In the abdominopelvic examination, her abdomen was flat and moved with respiration. She had a Pfannenstiel incision scar on the abdomen. There was no tenderness elicited and no organomegaly. Her bowel sounds were normoactive. She had normal genitalia with no lesions, no protrusions, and no discharge.

Examination of the central nervous system showed she was conscious, alert, and well-oriented. There was no sign of meningeal irritation or cranial nerve deficit. Her motor and sensory systems were normal. In her cardiovascular system, her pulse rate was 68 beats per minute, regular and of normal volume. Her blood pressure was 110/80mmHg; the apex beat was at the fifth left intercostal space, on the midclavicular line. Only the first and second heart sounds were heard. Examination of other systems revealed normal findings.

Assessment:

The assessment made was the need for bilateral tubal ligation reversal.

Management:

The client was made to understand what bilateral tubal ligation involved. She was told that it was a surgical procedure where a woman's fallopian tubes are permanently blocked or removed, thereby preventing fertilization of eggs by sperm and resultant conception.

Thus, it was an irreversible contraceptive method. She was then asked to perform a hysterosalpingogram (HSG) to ascertain the status of her fallopian tubes. She was scheduled for a second visit two days later.

Second visit:

At her second visit two days later, she had the result of the hysterosalpingogram. It showed a well-defined uterus with smooth contours. There was a filling of the proximal aspect of the fallopian tubes with an abrupt termination at the distal portion.

This result was carefully explained to the patient. She was gently informed that she could not become pregnant through regular sexual intercourse with her spouse. However, there were other options available for having more children. These included in-vitro fertilization, surrogacy, and adoption. A tubal reversal surgery could be done, but its success could not be guaranteed because of the extent of damage to the fallopian tubes due to the long duration of time since the procedure occurred. She was counseled to inform her husband and involve him in her decisions. The patient was visibly distressed and mentioned that she had not been informed about the irreversibility of the contraceptive method but was only told that it was the most effective way to avoid pregnancy. She was advised to discuss the issue with her husband and return with him in a week's time. A one-week appointment was scheduled.

Third visit:

She was seen a week later, accompanied by her husband. With her consent, the issues were discussed again with an enquiry made about their decisions.

Her husband said that though he was not happy knowing that her tubal ligation was irreversible, they were willing to attempt in-vitro fertilization. They were counseled on the cost, risks, benefits, and failure rates. Regarding the cost, the client was assured that her health insurance in Sweden could cover the procedure as she was desirous of having it done in Sweden, and as for the risks, she was prepared to do all she could to ensure the success of her marriage. They were both encouraged to support each other throughout the process. They agreed that they were happy with the counseling and decisions they had reached. Subsequently, the client was discharged from follow-up.

Summary:

A 42-year-old woman who had undergone a bilateral tubal ligation and desired to have it reversed because she had recently married a new husband. She was properly counselled on contraception and other reproduction options.

Discussion:

Family planning or contraception is unarguably one of the most important public health advancements in the last century. It can be defined as a woman's ability to decide if and when she wants to have children, including the number of children she chooses to have.[1] Statistics show that globally, 64% of women use a form of contraception, and more than 300 million people in 69 of the world's poorest countries use modern contraception.[1,2]

Different methods exist, which could be reversible or non-reversible. Female sterilization, which involves tubal ligation, is a permanent method of family planning. It involves a surgical procedure in which the fallopian tubes are permanently blocked or removed, thus impeding the fertilization of eggs by sperm and the subsequent implantation of a fertilized egg.[3,4] In this case study, the client had undergone a permanent method of family planning, tubal ligation, eight years earlier. Counselling for contraceptive methods involves empowering a client to make an informed decision.[5,6]

An informed choice encompasses knowledge of all available information relevant to the choice made, alternatives, advantages and disadvantages, and possible side effects. For irreversible methods, counseling should further discuss the permanence of the method, information about the surgical procedure, and the possibility of future regret.[5,6]

Regret after sterilization has been found to occur, with some women wanting to reverse the procedure. Studies have shown that as high as 20.3% of women 30 years or younger and 5.9% of those above 30 years expressed regret within 14 years of their tubal ligation.[3,7]

Important factors associated with regret include young age, unpredictable life events, desire for more children, change in marital status with a simultaneous desire to have more children with a new partner, and having few children at the time of sterilization.[4,7] This was the situation with this client, who had remarried after the death of her husband and wanted to have children with her new husband.

Regardless of the method that is being considered, reversible or irreversible, the goal of the clinician-patient dialogue is to ensure that the woman is properly counseled and given enough information and time to determine the best method for her at that point in her life.[8] In the case of sterilization, correct assessment should be made as to whether the woman has adequately considered the implications of ending her child-bearing potential.[9,10] Counselling must take into account each woman's knowledge base, cultural context, and experience. Proper counseling must consider the unique contraceptive history and contraceptive requirements of the client. As much as possible, wrong information or misperceptions should not be conveyed to the client. It was clear from the exchange that this client had not been properly counselled before the procedure to make an informed decision.

Lessons Learned/Recommendations:

Greater involvement of family physicians in family planning clinics is of utmost importance, being that this specialty appears to be the best equipped in counseling practices.

References

1. Daniels K, Abma JC. Current contraceptive status among women aged 15-49: United States, 2015-2017. NCHS Data Brief 2018: 327

2. ACOG Practice Bulletin No 208: Benefits and risks of sterilization. Obstetrics and Gynecology. March 2019; 133(3)

3. Shreffler KM, Greil AL, McQuillan J, Gallus KL. Reasons for tubal sterilization, regret and depressive symptoms. *J Reprod Infant Psychol.* 2016;34 (3):304–313

4. Borrero SB, Abebe K, Dehlendorf C, Schwarz EB. Racial variation in tubal sterilization rates: The role of patient-level factors. Fertility & Sterility. 2011; 95:17–22

5. Shreffler KM, McQuillan J, Greil AL, Johnson DR. Surgical sterilization, regret, and race: Contemporary patterns. Social Science Research. 2015; 50:31–45

6. Swende TZ, Hwande TS. Female sterilization by tubal ligation at caesarean section in Makurdi, Nigeria. Ann Afr Med. 2010; 9:246-50

7. Igberase GO, Ebeigbe PN, Umeora O, Abedi HO. Bilateral tubal ligation

8. Enyindah CE, Hassan KO, Ojule JD, Oranu EO. Knowledge and attitude of fertile women towards bilateral tubal ligation in Port Harcourt, Southern Nigeria. J Contracept Stud. 2018; 3(3):19

9. Chan LM, Westhoff CL. Tubal sterilization trends in the United States. Fertil Steril. 2010; 94:1

10. World Health Organization. Counselling for maternal and new-born healthcare: a handbook for building skills. Family Planning Counselling. 2013; 12

Chapter Twenty

The Effect Of Sexual Assault On The Family

This case revolved around three generations of a family and is presented in a unique way. It begins with the child as the central figure and then explores the ripple effects that manifest as medical conditions impacting the child's mother and grandmother. By examining the case in this order, we can see how the health issues affecting one family member can have a profound impact on others, illustrating the interconnectedness of family health dynamics.

Case 1: Genital injury due to sexual assault

A 2-year-old female child was brought to the clinic with complaints of pain and swelling of the vulva of approximately 2 hours' duration.

The patient was apparently well in the morning when her parents left for work. She was left in the care of a female domestic helper. When they returned, they noticed that she cried excessively and screamed anytime her mother tried to lift her up. Her mother also noticed that she was wearing a diaper which was contrary to the instruction she had given to her domestic help. The child was supposed to be off diapers in the daytime because she was being potty trained. She decided to examine her, and on removal of her diaper, she noticed that there was swelling of the child's vulva. The patient refused to allow her mother to touch her vulva due to pain. Her parents suspected that something bad had happened to her, but since she could not verbalize adequately and only cried, they only had a strong sense of suspicion. The domestic help denied having knowledge of the patient's condition.

On questioning the security man, they were told that the domestic help had received her brother, a 20-year-old man, who stayed for about four hours while the parents were at work and left approximately 2 hours before the child's parents returned home. He was an electrician and was well-known to the family for having done some repairs within the home. Her parents called the police, who arrested the domestic staff. Further questioning by the police revealed that while the nanny had been in the kitchen with the child sleeping in the living room, her brother had dug his fingers into her vagina, thereby injuring her.

He also tried to put his penis into her vagina but was unable to penetrate because it was so small. The domestic help was alerted by the child's cries. She tried to relieve her distress by using hot water to massage the genitalia, following which she attempted to conceal the act by putting a diaper on her and asking her brother to leave immediately. The police subsequently arrested the assailant, who stated that he did not have sexual intercourse with her but only put his fingers into the patient's genital and rubbed his penis on it. There was no fever, cough, abnormal pulling of the ears, swelling of any limb, or bleeding from the vagina.

Her parents, however, felt that he was lying and had had intercourse with her, hence the pain and swelling. They had an idea that Sexually Transmitted Infections (STIs), including Human Immunodeficiency Virus (HIV), could be transmitted through sexual exposure. Their fear was the possibility that the assailant might be infected with HIV or other STIs thereby infecting their daughter. They expected that she would be tested for HIV and STIs and given antiretroviral drugs.

The patient's past medical and surgical history showed that she had never been admitted to a health facility for any illness.

In the pregnancy, birth, and development history, it was seen that her pregnancy was planned, and she was born at term through spontaneous vaginal delivery at a hospital in the United States of America. Her birth weight was 3.3kg, and the pregnancy had been uneventful. Her developmental milestones were normal for her age.

The immunization and nutrition history showed she had received the complete immunization for her age evidenced by her immunization card and BCG scar on her left upper arm. She was exclusively fed breast milk in the first 3 months of life and was currently eating regular family meals.

In the family and social history, it was seen that the patient was the only child of her parents. Her mother was a 30-year-old accountant working at a commercial bank, while her father was a 37-year-old senior management staff at a construction company. They lived in a rented three-bedroom apartment and had three domestic staff. The family was at the early childbearing stage, according to the Evelyn Duvall model of family staging. Their source of healthcare finance was out-of-pocket. The physical examination revealed the patient as a healthy-looking girl who was afebrile, not pale, not jaundiced, not cyanosed, and with no significant peripheral lymphadenopathy or pedal oedema.

Her weight was 12.2kg, height 89cm, and occipital-frontal circumference 48cm, all of which were adequate for age. She was not wearing the same clothes she had on when the incident occurred.

Abdominopelvic examination showed the abdomen was full, soft, and moved with respiration. There was no tenderness elicited and no organ enlargement. Inspection of the anogenital region was done with the child in 3 positions: supine, knee-chest, and lateral decubitus positions. There was no discharge on the vulva or vagina, no lesions, and no vaginal protrusions. The labia were slightly oedematous and tender. There was a tender erythematous clitoris having a small cut. There was an intact hymen. Anal hygiene was good, and there were no lesions, protrusions, or bleeding from the anus. Anal and vaginal palpations were not done.

The central nervous system examination showed a conscious, alert, and irritable child. There were no signs of meningeal irritation or cranial nerve deficits. There was normal tone, power, and reflexes in all limbs. The patient's pulse rate was 120 beats per minute, with a regular rhythm and moderate volume. The first and second heart sounds were heard. In the respiratory system examination, the respiratory rate was 22 cycles per minute, chest expansion was equal, and she had good air entry in the lung fields. Her breath sounds were vesicular. Examination of the ears and nose did not yield any abnormalities. The throat examination showed normal palate, tonsils and fauces.

A provisional diagnosis of Genital Injury secondary to sexual assault was made.

Management:

The patient's diagnosis and management plan were explained to her parents. Laboratory investigations which included vaginal swab microscopy, culture and sensitivity (m/c/s), Venereal Disease Research Laboratory (VDRL) test, HIV screening and Hepatitis C virus screening would be done. When done, the results showed that HIV, Hepatitis C virus screening, and VDRL test were non-reactive. A request for HIV screening of the assailant was sent to the police, and they responded that it would be done after due administrative procedure. A forensic examination for semen was not done because there was no facility for it in the state. She was placed on Syrup Cefuroxime at a dose of 10mg/kg (5mls) twice daily for 7 days, Syrup Ibuprofen 5mls twice daily for 3 days and Syrup Vitamin C 5mls twice daily for a week. It was decided that she should commence post-exposure prophylaxis (PEP) since the retroviral status of the assailant was not known, and it was not certain when he would be screened. Her parents were asked to return with her the next day.

First follow-up visit:

When seen at her scheduled appointment, the parents were informed about the risks of Highly Active Antiretroviral Therapy (HAART), and they consented to commencing the drugs. Thus, she was given tablet Combivir (Zidovudine 300mg/Lamivudine 150mg) daily orally for a month according to her weight. HIV screening was to be repeated at 6 weeks, 3 months, and 6 months. A follow-up visit was scheduled in a week's time.

Second follow-up visit:

At this visit, her parents complained that she cried a lot and had experienced one episode of vomiting when she commenced the antiretroviral drugs. Her vital signs were normal. There was no complaint of abnormal vaginal discharge, and an examination of the genitalia revealed a normal vulva. The vaginal swab culture did not yield any isolated organisms. The incident had negatively affected their family life, and her two grandmothers had taken up temporary residence in their home to give psychological support to the family. Her mother complained of difficulty in sleeping, restlessness, and fatigue since the incident occurred, and she was counselled to rest adequately. She also complained of numerous conflicts with the patient's father as he blamed her for their child's predicament. Due to all the issues raised, the physician was concerned about the problems generated in this family due to the assault and thus set up a family conference to which the parents consented.

Family conference:

The family conference was convened two days after the previous visit. It was held at the hospital consulting room and was attended by the child's parents, grandmothers, and maternal aunt. The assault incident, the effects of the assault on the family, the prosecution of the assailant, and the way forward after the assault event were discussed. Her parents were encouraged not to be anxious over the possibility of the patient acquiring HIV as it had been found that there was no vaginal penetration, evidenced by her intact hymen. The HIV screening of the assailant was negative, and it helped to relieve some of their anxiety. The author counseled the family on the importance of rendering mutual support to themselves to aid the healing process. It would also prevent family dysfunction and medical issues like hypertension. She also suggested a change of environment as well as a change of domestic staff ,which the patient's father affirmed had already been done. The maternal grandmother had decided to stay with them until she was enrolled in nursery school. Follow-up was scheduled for a month after the conference.

Third follow-up visit:

At this visit, the patient had completed her antiretroviral medication, and she was in a normal state of health. The HIV test was non-reactive. Subsequently, she was seen three and six months after the initial presentation, both times in the company of her parents. She was in a good state of health. The HIV tests were non-reactive. She had also been enrolled in a nursery school and was adjusting well.

Case 2: Mother

Generalized Anxiety Disorder

A 30-year-old woman presented with excessive worry, restlessness, and sleep disturbance of 7 months duration

The patient was apparently well until about 7 months before her visit, when it was observed that she worried excessively. This started gradually but progressively became worse over the previous three months. About eight months before the presentation, her young child had been the victim of a sexual assault, and she was constantly worrying even though her daughter had been treated and was in a stable state. Most times, she would imagine that her daughter would be assaulted again, and she found it difficult to control her worried state. There was also the recurrent inability to initiate and maintain sleep at night. On most nights, she would stay awake till the early hours of the morning, even during her work week. She usually slept for only 2-3 hours whenever she fell asleep. Therefore, she was usually fatigued at work and would fall asleep at odd hours. This led to her having queries at work from her superiors. Her concentration was impaired, and she occasionally complained of palpitations. There was no associated irritability, excessive sweating, weight loss, heat intolerance, diarrhea, tremors, low mood, low energy, or feeling of worthlessness. There was no history of suicidal ideation, visual or auditory hallucinations, loss of interest in pleasurable activities, frequent urination, increased thirst, headache, or blurring of vision. She occasionally took Phenergan tablets to help her sleep. She did not indulge in alcohol, tobacco, or illicit substances. Her source of hope was God, and she belonged to an organized religious group. Her spiritual belief did not stop her from seeking medical care. She initially thought that these symptoms were due to pregnancy, but upon doing a pregnancy test, which turned out negative, she decided to seek medical intervention. She now felt that her symptoms were due to work stress. The illness had affected her work as well as her devotion to the care of her family, as her husband stated that she was always tired. She expected to receive medications that would make her feel relaxed.

Her past medical and surgical history showed she was not a known hypertensive, diabetic, asthmatic, or sickle cell disease patient. Her only hospital admission was during childbirth. She was not on any routine drugs and had no known drug allergy.

She had her first menstrual flow at 11 years. Her menstrual periods lasted for 5 days, and the cycle length was 28 days. She was $P1.^{+0}$

There was no history of dysmenorrhea or menorrhagia, and she occasionally used barrier contraception (condoms). She was the third of three children, two females, and one male. Her parents were alive. Her mother was known to be hypertensive. APGAR score assessment of her family was 7/10 portraying a moderately dysfunctional family. The family's source of finance for healthcare was out-of-pocket.

The general physical examination revealed a young woman who was well-dressed and anxious-looking as evidenced by an inability to sit still. She was well-oriented in time, place and person. She was afebrile (temperature 37.1^0 C), not pale, not cyanosed, not jaundiced, and with no peripheral lymphadenopathy or pedal oedema. She was 1.64 metres tall, weighed 62 kg, and her body mass index was $23.05 kg/m^2$, which was adequate.

A mini-mental state examination was done and revealed a score of 28/30 (orientation-10, registration-3, attention, and calculation-4, recall-3, and language-8), showing that there was no cognitive impairment. Generalized Anxiety Disorder -7 assessment showed a score of 10, indicating moderate anxiety disorder.

Examination of the neck showed no swellings and no tenderness. Examination of the central nervous system indicated that there was no sign of meningeal irritation and no cranial nerve deficit. There was no motor or sensory deficit. An examination of the eyes showed no swellings or discharge. Visual acuity was normal (6/6), pupils reacted normally to light, and she had a normal cup-disc ratio.

Her respiratory rate was 22 cycles per minute, and the chest was clinically clear. The patient's pulse rate was 94 beats per minute with a full volume and regular rhythm. Her blood pressure was 110/80 mmHg; jugular venous pressure was not raised, and the apex beat was located at the 5th left intercostal space on the Mid-clavicular line. The first and second heart sounds were heard.

Diagnosis:

A diagnosis of moderate generalized anxiety disorder was made. Differential diagnoses included depression and panic disorder.

Management:

The patient's diagnosis and possible risk factors were explained to her. It was explained to her that the most likely risk factor in her case was the family stressor due to her daughter's assault incident. The importance of family support was emphasized, and her husband was counselled to continue supporting her and also ensure that she adhered to her medication. The investigations included urinalysis and thyroid function test. The results showed normal parameters. Her management plan included medications and psychotherapy. The medications prescribed for her included tablet sertraline 25 mg daily orally for 2 weeks, tablets bromazepam 3 mg nocte orally for 4 days, and then 1.5 mg nocte orally for 3 days. She was enlightened on the side effects of the drugs. She was co-managed with the clinical psychologist who administered cognitive behavioural therapy on her. She was given two-week sick leave to rest adequately, commence her medications and attend CBT sessions. She was given a one-week follow-up appointment.

One week follow-up visit:

She attended her follow-up appointment in company of her husband. There were no new complaints, and she was taking her medications. She was calmer but still worried occasionally. Her sleeping pattern had improved, and she felt more refreshed. Bromazepam was discontinued from her drugs and sertraline was continued for 2 months. She was subsequently scheduled for follow-up visits once a month for the next 3 months. She was also encouraged to keep her appointments with the clinical psychologist.

Other follow-up visits:

At each visit, she was counselled to get adequate rest, regular exercise, good nutrition, participation in activities pleasurable to her, and maintain positive spirituality, as she was a devout Christian. GAD-7 tool was used at each follow-up visit to monitor her response to her management and she showed satisfactory response.

Case 3: Grandmother

Severe Hypertension

A 62-year-old woman presented at the clinic with a headache and dizziness of 1 week duration.

She had a known hypertensive diagnosed seven years earlier. She presented with a headache, which was of insidious onset, located on the temporal regions, throbbing in nature, relieved by analgesics, and aggravated by the mobility of the head and noise. There was no history of fever, vomiting, trauma to the head, neck stiffness, or seizures.

Dizziness was gradual in onset, relieved by rest and aggravated by movement. There was associated difficulty in initiating sleep as the patient found it difficult to sleep well due to headaches.

There was no history of loss of consciousness, ear pain or trauma, urinary symptoms, cough, palpitations, or chest pain. Her routine drugs were Amlodipine, Normoretic, and Vasoprin, but in the past three months, she had not adhered to her antihypertensive medications because she was occupied with taking care of her young granddaughter, who had suffered a sexual assault and supporting her daughter through the ordeal. She had not attended her follow-up visits for a while because she was out of her usual location. The patient felt that her symptoms were due to malaria, which had been triggered by stress. She did not have any fears concerning her illness, and she expected to be treated for malaria and have her blood pressure checked.

In the past medical and surgical history, there was no known history of diabetes, asthma, epilepsy, or sickle cell disease. There was no history of surgery or blood transfusion. There was no history of allergy to any drugs. She was Para 3^{+0} (all alive), her menarche was at the age of 14 years, and she was about eleven years post-menopausal. She had used Billing's method of contraception before she became menopausal. There was no history of abnormal vaginal bleeding, abdominal pain or breast masses. Her last Pap smear was five years earlier.

The patient was the fourth child in a family of 8 children (4 males and four females). All her siblings were alive, but both parents were deceased through natural causes. There was a family history of hypertension and diabetes, as her two sisters had hypertension and her brother had diabetes. She was an entrepreneur involved in estate management and venture capitalism. She was married to a 68-year-old lawyer who owned a law firm. They had three children, two females and one male, aged 36, 33 and 30 years. They were all married with children. She lived with her husband in a six-bedroom home in Lagos. However, at the time of her visit, she was living in her daughter's home in Calabar. Her family stage was middle-aged family (Evelyn Duvall's stage 7). Apgar's assessment of her family was 10/10, showing a highly functional family.

The general physical examination revealed an elderly woman who was healthy-looking and well-kempt. She was not febrile, not pale, not jaundiced, not dehydrated, and did not have significant peripheral lymphadenopathy or pedal oedema. Her weight was 72kg, height 1.65 metres, and she had a body mass index of $25.97 kg/m^2$, indicating that she was overweight. She was well-oriented in time, place and person. There were no neurological deficits detected in her.

Examination of the eyes showed her visual acuity to be 6/6 in both eyes. The ophthalmoscopic examination was normal with no evidence of arterio-venous thickening or presence of exudates.

The patient's pulse rate was 64 beats per minute, with a regular rhythm and normal volume. There was synchrony of her radial pulse with other peripheral pulses. Her blood pressure was 180/110 mmHg, jugular venous pressure was not raised, and the apex beat was on the fifth left intercostal space at the mid-clavicular line. The first and second heart sounds were only auscultated.

Her respiratory rate was 16 cycles per minute. The trachea was central, with symmetrical chest movement and resonant percussion notes. Air entry was good in all lung fields, and breath sounds were vesicular. Abdominal examination showed her abdomen was full, with no areas of tenderness and no palpable organomegaly. Bowel sounds were heard and were normal. Musculoskeletal system examination showed normal tone, power, and reflexes in all limbs.

A diagnosis of Severe Hypertension in a non-adherent patient was made.

Management:

The diagnosis and management plan were explained to the patient. She was educated that her symptoms were due to an acute rise in her blood pressure due to non-adherence to her therapy. She was made to understand that non-adherence could result in complications even for a patient who had been on regular medication and thus advised to adhere to her medication always regardless of any pressures she may be facing. The risk factors, including the positive family history of hypertension and diabetes, were discussed, and she was advised on the Dietary Approach to Stop Hypertension (DASH) diet. She was counselled on the need for regular monitoring of her blood pressure with her own personal kit at home and regular medical check-ups.

The investigations that were done included blood film for malaria parasite, urinalysis, fasting lipid profile (FLP), fasting blood glucose (FBG), and assay for electrolytes, urea, and creatinine (EUC), and chest x-ray. The results were as follows: blood film for malaria parasites showed scanty trophozoites of malaria parasites; FBG was 3.8mmol/l; FLP, urinalysis, and EUC showed normal parameters. The chest radiograph showed unfolding of the aorta, which indicated long-standing hypertension.

She was given oral tablets of Nifedipine 20 mg daily, 1 tablet of Amiloride/ hydrochlorothiazide daily, and Bromazepam 1.5 mg daily, all for one week. She was also given oral tablets of Arthemether/Lumefantrine 80/480 mg twice daily for three days. She was advised to rest adequately and given a one-week follow-up appointment.

One week follow-up:

She did not have any complaints and had taken all her medications. Her blood pressure was 140/80 mmHg. She was made to continue with tablets of Amlodipine 10 mg daily and 1 tablet Amiloride/ hydrochlorothiazide daily for one month.

A one-month follow-up appointment was scheduled.

One-month follow-up:

When seen one month later, she had no new complaints. She was adhering to her medications. Her blood pressure was 130/80 mmHg, and her weight was 71 kg. Subsequently, she was given monthly follow-up visits and advised to continue that way even when she returned to her permanent location.

FAMILY GENOGRAM

Date created: 8/8/17
Last updated: 15/11/19

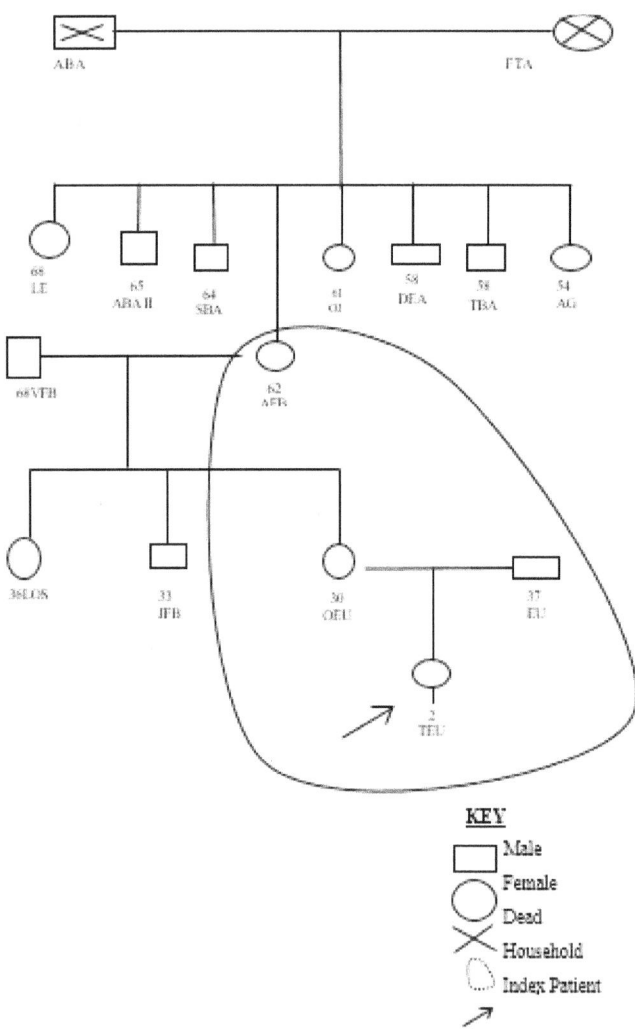

DISCUSSION

The family is the fundamental unit of any society and constitutes a major factor that can influence the well-being and development of individuals. Family health is thus an important aspect of individual health as it can influence the causation of disease and determine therapeutic success or failure. In this family case study, there was a portrayal of how the disease of one member of a family strongly impacted the causation of diseases in other family members.

The index patient was a very young female child who was sexual assaulted by an adult man who was her caregiver's brother, and this assault resulted in genital injury. Child sexual assault or abuse is the involvement of children and adolescents in sexual activities that they cannot fully comprehend or consent to as equal participants.[1] A meta-analysis of 323 studies from around the world showed an overall prevalence of 12.7% (18% for girls and 7.6% for boys).[2] Data from Nigeria is sparse because many cases go unreported due to the stigma attached. The spectrum can range from non-invasive activities where there is no physical contact to brutal encounters such as rape.[1]

Sexual assault could present with genital injury such as abrasions, cuts, swellings in the genitalia, hymen tears, and vaginal bleeding.[1,3] In this case, the findings seen in the index patient were vulva swelling and vulva pain possibly caused by cuts and abrasions from the assailant's nails. Sometimes, positive findings on physical examination may be rare, and this may be adduced to the frequently long interval between abuse and physical examination, absence of physical injuries, and the inability of the child to complain or verbalize the symptoms due to factors like young age and fear.[1] The inability to report the exact details of the assault was an important challenge in the management of this 2-year old patient as her speech was not fully developed. Thus, a thorough physical examination with a high level of suspicion was done.

A comprehensive treatment of sexual assault must address issues like physical injuries, pregnancy, STIs, HIV, Hepatitis B, counseling and social support.[3,4] Physical injuries, if present, should be appropriately treated. The index patient had injuries in the vulva. It is recommended that patients should be tested for chlamydia, gonorrhoea, trichomoniasis, syphilis, HIV, and hepatitis B on a case-by-case basis.[4] In the index patient, screenings for syphilis, HIV, and Hepatitis C virus were done due to genital examination findings as well as to allay the fears of the parents. Due to the possibility of acquiring an infectious disease, it has been recommended that providers should administer appropriate therapy to prevent this transmission.[3] For this reason, this patient was given prophylactic broad-spectrum antibiotics. In addition, post-exposure prophylaxis should be carefully explained to patients with its risks and benefits. After consultation with her parents, the index patient was administered post-exposure prophylaxis, and this helped to calm her parent's fears.

Studies have revealed an association between sexual assault and negative health effects which could impact families.[3] The incident caused such psychological distress in the index patient's mother that she developed generalized anxiety disorder.

Generalized anxiety disorder is a mental illness that is characterized by persistent and excessive worry about different things.[5] Patients with this disorder usually anticipate disaster and may be overly concerned over family, money, health, work, interpersonal relationships, and other issues.[5] Other symptoms include restlessness, easy fatigue, sleep disturbances, and muscle tension.[6,7] The index patient's mother presented with excessive worry and sleep disturbance, which had even affected her work, leading to poor work performance.

Some factors found to increase the risk of generalized anxiety disorder include genetic predisposition, substance use, low socioeconomic status, old age, disrupted family environments, and sexual abuse. The risk factor that was seen in the index patient's mother was the sexual abuse of her daughter. Management of generalized anxiety disorder involves psychotherapy and pharmacotherapy.[7] She was managed with psychotherapy and selective serotonin reuptake inhibitors such as paroxetine, as well as Bromazepam, a benzodiazepine. Other treatment measures include lifestyle factors such as stress management, stress reduction, relaxation techniques, and exercise.[6,7]

In the process of caring for her daughter and young granddaughter in their period of distress, the grandmother who was known to hypertensive neglected to take her antihypertensive drugs, and this resulted in severe hypertension. Management of the grandmother placed emphasis on medication adherence,[8,9,10] and this produced positive outcomes. As part of the interventions given to this family, a family conference was carried out. This was aimed at assisting them in their healing process as well as to prevent family dysfunction known to be a common sequel in such incidents.[3]

Lessons Learned/Recommendations:

This case portrayed the cycle of illness conditions that could occur in a family following a sexual assault incident. It explored the interconnected health issues of a three-generation family, highlighting the far-reaching impact of family health dynamics.

There is a need for primary care physicians to pay close attention to the holistic management of victims of sexual assault and their families including mental health care and social support.

References

1. Gallion HR, Milam LJ, Littrel LL. Genital findings in cases of child sexual abuse: genital versus vaginal penetration. Journal of paediatric and adolescent gynecology. 2016; 29(6): 604-611

2. Stoltenborgh M, van Ijzendoorn MH, Euser EM, Bakermans-Kranenburg MJ. A global perspective on child sexual abuse: Meta-analysis of prevalence around the world. Child Maltreat. 2011; 16:79–101.

3. Herrmann B, Banaschak S, Csorba R, Navratil F, Dettmeyer R. Physical Examination in Child Sexual Abuse: Approaches and Current Evidence. *Deutsches Ärzteblatt International*. 2014; 111(41):692-703.

4. David N, Ezechi O, Wapmuk A, Gbajabiamila T, Ohihoin A, Herbertson E, et al. Child sexual abuse and

disclosure in Southwestern Nigeria: a community based study. *Afr Health Sci.* 2018;18(2):199–208.

5. Okeke T, Anyaehie U, Ezenyeaku C. An overview of female genital mutilation in Nigeria. Annals of Medical and Health Sciences Research. 2012; 2(1):70-73.

6. Abdulkadir I, Umar LW, Musa HH, Musa S, Oyeniyi OA, Ayoola-Williams OM, Okeniyi L. Child sexual abuse: A review of cases seen at General Hospital Suleja, Niger State. Ann Nigerian Med 2011; 5:15-9

7. Somoye EB, Babalola EO, Adebowale TO. Prevalence and risk factors for anxiety and depression among commercial bank workers in Abeokuta, South-west Nigeria. J Behav Health. 2015; 4:201-9

8. Bhattacharya D, Tk S, Lyle N, Jana U, Pk D. A clinical study on the management of generalized anxiety disorder with Vaca (Acorus calamus). Indian J Tradit Knowl. 2011;10(4):668-71

9. Plummer F, Manea L, Trepel D, McMillan D. Screening for anxiety disorders with the GAD-7 and GAD-2: a systematic review and diagnostic meta-analysis. Gen Hosp Psychiatry. 2016; 39:24-31.

10. Badru OA, Ogunlesi AO, Ogunwale A, Abdulmalik JO, Yusuf OB. Prevalence of generalized anxiety disorder and major depression among correctional officers in a Nigerian prison. The Journal of Forensic Psychiatry & Psychology. 2018: 29(4):509-526

11. Adisa R, Ilesanmi OA, Fakeye TO. Treatment adherence and blood pressure outcome among hypertensive out-patients in two tertiary hospitals in Sokoto, Northwestern Nigeria. *BMC Cardiovasc Disord.* 2018; 18(1):194

12. Brown MT, Bussell JK. Medication adherence: WHO cares? Mayo Clin Proc 2011; 86:304–14

13. Akintunde A, Akintunde T. Antihypertensive medications adherence among Nigerian hypertensive

subjects in a specialist clinic compared to a general outpatient clinic. Annals of Medical and Health Sciences Research. 2015; 5(3):173-178.

14. Najimi A, Mostafavi F, Sharifirad G, Golshiri P. Barriers to medication adherence in patients with hypertension: A qualitative study. *J Educ Health Promot.* 2018; 7:24.

15. Ogunkoya OE, Besidonne CE. A review of the DASH plan in Nigeria. J Pub Health Catalog 2019;2(2):156-16

Index

Allergic conjunctivitis in a primary school child   4-11

External hordeolum in a make-up artist   12-19

Recurrent pelvic inflammatory disease in a 28-year-old woman with multiple sexual partners   20-28

Septic abortion in a teenager   29-37

Malaria in pregnancy   38-45

Retained placenta in a housewife   46-53

Foreign body in the ear   54-61

Chronic leg ulcer in a female traffic warden   62-70

Left dorsal ganglion cyst   71-77

Severe hypertension due to poor adherence   78-86

Urinary tract infection in a 33-year-old housewife with ectopic kidney   87-94

Food poisoning in a 36-year-old nurse   95-101

Vaso-occlusive crisis in a 7-year-old child   102-109

Scabies in a 13-year-old secondary school student   110-117

Acute pharyngitis in a 10-year-old boy   117-124

Cervical spondylosis in a 70-year-old pensioner   124-131

Depression in a 43-year-old welder with burns injury   132-139

Post-traumatic stress disorder following intimate partner violence   140-147

Importance of adequate counselling in family planning clinic   148-154

The effect of sexual assault on the family   155-172

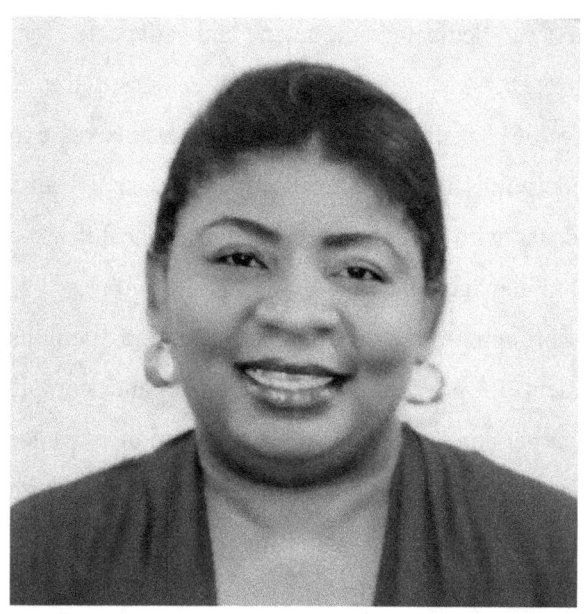

About the Author

Dr. Queeneth Adams is a seasoned family physician with over two decades of clinical experience. She earned her medical degree from the prestigious University of Calabar and later became a Fellow of the National Postgraduate Medical College of Nigeria, specializing in Family Medicine.

Dr. Adams' passion for global health and leadership led her to pursue further education in the United States, where she earned an MSc in Global Health Policy and Management from Brandeis University, Massachusetts, and an MBA from Anna Maria College, Massachusetts.

As a dedicated clinician and advocate for quality healthcare, Dr. Adams is an active member of the American Academy of Family Physicians. Her extensive experience, combined with her advanced education and training, has equipped her with a unique perspective on healthcare delivery, policy, and management.

Throughout her career, Dr. Adams has demonstrated a commitment to providing compassionate and comprehensive care to her patients while also contributing to the advancement of healthcare systems and policies. Her expertise and insights make her a valuable voice in the medical community, and her writing offers a wealth of knowledge and experience to readers.

www.ingramcontent.com/pod-product-compliance
Lightning Source LLC
Chambersburg PA
CBHW052237220526
45471CB00001B/81